T0074124

ALL BLEEDING STOPS

ALL
BLEEDING
STOPS

LIFE and DEATH
in the
TRAUMA UNIT

STEPHEN M. COHN, M.D.

MAYO CLINIC PRESS
200 First St. SW
Rochester, MN 55905
mcpress.mayoclinic.org

To stay informed about Mayo Clinic Press, please subscribe to our free e-newsletter at
mcpress.mayoclinic.org or follow us on social media.

For bulk sales to employers, member groups and health-related companies, contact Mayo
Clinic at SpecialSalesMayoBooks@mayo.edu.

Proceeds from the sale of every book benefit important medical research and education at
Mayo Clinic.

Cover design by Nikolaas Eickelbeck

Library of Congress Cataloging-in-Publication Data

Names: Cohn, Stephen M., author.
Title: All bleeding stops : life and death in the trauma unit / Stephen M. Cohn.
Description: First edition. | Rochester, MN : Mayo Clinic Press, 2023. |
    Includes bibliographical references.
Identifiers: LCCN 2023006599 (print) | LCCN 2023006600 (ebook) | ISBN
    9798887700632 (hardcover) | ISBN 9798887700649 (epub)
Subjects: MESH: Trauma Centers | Surgeons—psychology | Emergencies |
    United States
Classification: LCC RA645.5 (print) | LCC RA645.5 (ebook) | NLM WX 215 |
    DDC 362.18—dc23/eng/20230703
LC record available at https://lccn.loc.gov/2023006599
LC ebook record available at https://lccn.loc.gov/2023006600

Printed in the U.S.A.

First edition: 2023

"A new truth does not triumph by convincing its opponents . . . but rather because they eventually die."
Max Planck, 1858–1947

In memory of Lee and Iris, and Rosie who instilled in me a sense of unlimited possibility.

To Miryame, Sam, Liz, and Claudia, who encouraged me to write this book and whose love and guidance made the journey worthwhile.

To my current and former colleagues and trainees, brothers and sisters in the field, who continue to meet the challenges and save lives.

CONTENTS

ALL BLEEDING STOPS

INTRODUCTION

*We always say, "All bleeding stops." And it's a true statement,
one way or another. . . . It distills into a few words the battle we
trauma surgeons fight each and every day.*

Eddie was on his way to high school on a blue-sky morning.
Then he was bleeding to death in front of me, lying on the
operating table with his belly open and filled with blood. He had
been an unbelted passenger thrown from the pickup truck he was
riding in when struck broadside by (I later learned) a drunk driver.
But at this point I wasn't thinking about that. I was operating on
this young man's abdomen, and there was massive bleeding coming from behind the liver whenever I lessened pressure. With my
left hand, I squeezed upward on the undersurface of the liver,
while with my right hand I compressed the aorta (the main arterial blood vessel to the abdomen) down into the spine. If I applied
too much pressure on the liver, I would cut off the blood returning
to the heart; not enough, and the abdomen would flood again
with blood. I was running out of hands.

The anesthesia team was frantically trying to keep up with the
hemorrhage, transfusing pint after pint of blood. Fortunately, a
transplant surgeon who saw the commotion and sensed we could

use some help provided a much-needed additional pair of hands. We managed to stem the torrent of blood by repairing a huge vein gushing from behind Eddie's liver and placing some large gauze packs into his abdomen. Eddie's life was hanging by the proverbial thread. We had stemmed the flow of blood in his abdomen, but anesthesia reported that blood was now pouring out through his breathing tube and that his oxygen levels were dangerously low despite maximal support. It was clear that he had a major lung injury. A critical decision had to be made. In that instant, I did not have the luxury of time to consider that this could be one of my own teenagers (who had also driven to school that morning). There was no time to reflect on the gravity of the situation or empathize with Eddie's family, who would be devastated by the loss of their young son with his entire life ahead of him.

To slow the hemorrhage from Eddie's lungs, I decided to abort the operation and take him immediately to the angiography suite, where our interventional radiologists could try using balloon catheter occlusion. (These are thin plastic catheters inserted into the bloodstream with a tiny inflatable balloon at the tip of the catheter that can narrow or dilate a blood vessel.) Imagine a large entourage of healthcare providers navigating carefully through the hospital's hallways, pushing a dying seventeen-year-old and a stretcher loaded with monitors while bagging the patient (manually squeezing in air through his breathing tube) and pouring fluids into him as a trail of blood splashes onto the ground. Eddie's heart stopped multiple times in radiology, but we were able to restore his circulation each time. He barely survived to reach the intensive care unit (ICU).

Throughout all this seeming mayhem, the trauma surgeon in charge (me, in this case) had to conduct a sort of symphony involving a complex team of healthcare providers in multiple disciplines. I had to coordinate and anticipate all needed lifesaving events for this young man, even as I did not (and could not) fully understand the magnitude of all his injuries. In a case like this, survival depends on a combination of knowledge, instinct, resources, and, alas, good fortune. I had to remain calm throughout this process, focusing solely on the challenge at hand and quickly recalibrating my interventions based on the responses of the patient. Trauma surgeons do not have time to methodically calculate the risks and benefits of each decision. We must trust our training and experience to make instantaneous, critical, and, hopefully, correct decisions.

All afternoon, we worked relentlessly on Eddie in the ICU with a team of about twenty-five doctors, nurses, pharmacists, and respiratory therapists. Despite our best efforts, the patient was still losing a tremendous amount of blood. Blood bank personnel provided a continuous stream of blood and plasma. We used a cell saver device, which cleaned the liters of blood pouring out of his abdomen and chest and reinfused them into his body. Each time we tried to employ the ventilator, the pressure within his chest was so high that the machine would malfunction, and Eddie's heart would stop. To counter this, medical students took turns bagging the patient. We define a "massive" transfusion as 10 units of blood (about 3.5 liters; a complete blood volume is 5.5 liters) in twenty-four hours. This amount of blood infusion is only required in a tiny fraction of trauma admissions. In this case, we infused Eddie with over 550 units of red blood cells, plus liters of his recycled blood, more than 35 entire blood volumes (about 200 liters) in all. (This may be the Guinness record for a trauma case. My next-highest transfusion volume in a trauma survivor was approximately 150 units, or 53 liters, in about one hour.)

At least three or four times during this eight-hour period, I was able to catch a few minutes to sit with Eddie's mother in the waiting area to tell her that we were trying everything. All too frequently, our communication with family during cardiopulmonary resuscitation (CPR) is followed by another appearance with the sad news that the patient has passed away. But amazingly, we were able to restore Eddie's circulation each time. As I left his mother sobbing in the family area, I felt her eyes following me. I knew what I would want if this were one of my kids. Press on! Then, for some inexplicable reason, Eddie stopped bleeding. Perhaps some of his mother's prayers were answered. We were all astonished by what seemed like a miracle.

But Eddie's lungs still were not functioning. I had spoken with the cardiothoracic team shortly after the patient arrived and asked them to stand by. So when we stabilized Eddie, they put him on the heart bypass circuit called extracorporeal membrane oxygenation (ECMO). This process allows us to load oxygen into the blood as it passes through a machine outside of the body, so functioning lungs are not required. Success! We returned to the operating room the next day to repair injuries not addressed during the first evaluation. After four days on the bypass circuit, Eddie's lungs improved. He ultimately survived and walked out of the hospital months later. Amazingly, Eddie finished high school on time. I am sure this young man has no concept of what an incredible collaborative effort it took to save his life. And how could he? How can anyone who is not intimately involved in such efforts?

And yet, the trauma team's response to Eddie's fantastic "save" was not one of joy and popping champagne bottles or even high-fiving with the other healthcare providers. Rather, it was a sober recognition that his survival was related to the proximity of his vehicle crash to a major trauma center replete with an experienced trauma team and awash in enormous resources. We have an expression in surgery that I abhor: "Better lucky than good." I would never want my survival or that of my family to depend on good fortune. Add to that the frustration that this entire near-tragic scenario could have been avoided if Eddie had been wearing a seat belt or if that drunk driver had not been on the road. According to the National Highway Traffic Safety Administration (NHTSA), nearly half of the passenger vehicle occupants killed annually are not wearing seat belts. Wearing a seat belt keeps you in the vehicle. The likelihood of a significant injury or death is much higher if you are flying out the window of a moving vehicle. Driving while under the influence is certainly preventable and, according to the Centers for Disease Control and Prevention (CDC), accounts for almost one-third of vehicle-related deaths each year. Perhaps an initial solution is as simple as providing vehicles with an ignition system that requires occupants to employ their seat belts and drivers to exhale into a breathalyzer before starting the engine.

Currently, the number of individuals seeking medical attention each year in US emergency departments for injuries exceeds one hundred million. Therefore, about one out of three Americans comes to the ER every year for some type of trauma. Yet not all trauma cases in an ER require a trauma surgeon. And not all trauma surgeons work many hours in the ER—in fact, most do not. Trauma surgeons are general surgeons, the jacks-of-all-trades, which means that we sometimes get a bad rap as the masters of nothing. In reality, however, trauma surgeons need to be experts at dealing with calamity. We are the tip of the spear, dealing with many of the catastrophic events that occur throughout a hospital: salvaging the woman bleeding to death during childbirth, inserting a tube into the trachea of a patient in the medical ICU when no one can get an airway, and assisting other surgeons in both the operating room and the ICU when their patients are critically ill. This, in addition to managing all the injured folks arriving at the trauma center and operating on patients with general surgical emergencies (like an inflamed appendix or gallbladder or anything bleeding, obstructed, or perforated). We are glue people, helping to hold together the entire hospital enterprise.

All Bleeding Stops will give readers a portrait of what we trauma surgeons do and explain our place in the US healthcare delivery system. I pull back the curtain on the field of trauma surgery, revealing insights that only a surgeon who has lived and breathed trauma for four decades can. There is art and science in the job, but the balance tips toward art in the conduct of trauma surgery—and surgery in general, in that both are based on experience more than high-quality science or scientific evidence. But where high-quality data exists, we aspire to use such information to guide our treatment.

All Bleeding Stops will also examine how societal attitudes and policies impact the deluge of injured patients we see every day—in other words, injury intervention and prevention. One frustrating aspect of trauma care is patients' lack of adherence to both good judgment and tried-and-true methods of avoiding devastating injury. A perfect example is the wearing of helmets. Helmets prevent serious brain injury and save lives, whether worn while riding a bicycle or a motorcycle. In 1976, states began to reduce and repeal helmet laws in response to Congress revoking federal authority to enforce penalties for noncompliance. As a result, there was a huge increase in severe head trauma cases after motorcycle crashes. You usually do not die when you crash your motorcycle while not wearing a helmet. But the head injury you sustain may prevent you from ever again performing the simple activities of daily living like eating, talking, or brushing your teeth. Unquestionably, our current societal norms and attitudes impact the likelihood of sustaining a severe injury. This discussion will help readers understand the connection between the laws we choose to enact, the behavior we choose to sanction, the everyday decisions we make, and the real-life, very personal consequences of those actions. The hope is that by improving awareness, we can prevent injury before it happens.

As a young surgeon, I found I could impart knowledge in a more meaningful and lasting way to my medical students and surgical residents by relating an experience to illustrate some essential points of information. Over the years, I have collected teaching narratives—experiences that are at times harrowing, at times tragic, and at times seemingly miraculous—all designed to drive home critical points in patient management. I am certainly not the authority on many of the topics covered here, but I am a senior surgeon with years of civilian and military surgical experience who naturally developed a particular perspective. The episodes recounted in this book come out of this experience. I focus on the impact of various injury mechanisms (blunt trauma such as vehicular crashes and falls, and penetrating injuries such as gunshot wounds and stab wounds), and I meticulously explore specific injuries to various parts of the body (the head, the chest, and the abdomen, for example). To understand how we take care of the severest of injuries, one must also understand how trauma systems and trauma centers work and how all the parts interrelate. The way we manage a trauma patient at the scene of a car crash in the United States differs from how it is done in other parts of the world. In Paris, France, for example, first responders employ a pre-hospital strategy based on the "stay and play" philosophy. This brings trauma resuscitation resources into the street. By contrast, in the United States, this care is typically provided in the emergency department of a hospital (so we "scoop and run").

At times, our dealings with patients and their families represent a microcosm of the challenges we encounter in interacting with society at large. The objective of the trauma team is to provide optimal patient care to achieve the best possible outcomes. However, trying to navigate the human equation of emotions inherent in each victim and their family members when faced with devastating injuries naturally is very difficult. When confronted with the impending loss of a loved one and a barrage of confusing new information, family members inevitably feel unhinged and out of control. I have heard people say that the stream of anonymous white jackets and the sterile, antiseptic environment of the trauma center make the uninitiated feel like they are in a swirling vortex without a stable surface on which to land.

One of the challenges in writing *All Bleeding Stops* was to convey some of the compassion of typical trauma providers. I say "challenges" because it can understandably appear that trauma providers display very little empathy for patients as people, as suffering human beings. More often, it might seem that we are problem-solvers. I suppose that the near-daily bombardment with self-induced or avoidable lunacy resulting in horrific injuries makes trauma surgeons (and probably the entire trauma team) numb to tragedy. People have often asked how a particular patient or patient event made me feel. The answer is that most trauma surgeons are not great "feelers." While I may tear up during emotional events in my life, at work these feelings are detrimental to optimal patient care when decisions must be made at a breakneck pace with no room for error. Perhaps trauma surgeons are made that way from the outset, or maybe we become hardened due to the catastrophes we must experience every day.

Trauma surgeons face challenges that are unique in the field of medicine. We have to deal with a steady diet of calamity; we face a dying trauma patient without any knowledge of the patient's underlying medical history, without knowing the actual injuries sustained, and without knowing the patient's and family's wishes. In *All Bleeding Stops*, I will explore the insanity trauma surgeons encounter, the obstacles to optimal care, and the frustration we must overcome to save lives.

1

WHAT EXACTLY IS A
TRAUMA SURGEON?

What is the difference between a trauma surgeon and a terrorist?
You can reason with a terrorist!
STEVE ROSS, M.D.

People have a strange fascination with the myriad foreign objects that surgeons fish out of the rectums of their patients. The end of the large intestine, the rectum, contains valves that help collect stool before evacuation. These valves also prevent the removal of foreign objects inserted in this location. So when an individual decides to place a can of hairspray, a champagne flute, or a vibrator (still vibrating) in the rectum, it can be challenging to retrieve. Therefore, it should have been no surprise when a senior resident called me during my chief residency year at the county hospital following an operation he performed to remove a massive cucumber from the rectum of a young male patient. When I asked why I was being honored with this lovely phone call, I was informed, "He's the salad chef at the Café Budapest," where I had dined the previous weekend.

The select group of general surgeons in the United States who specialize in the care of trauma patients is often confused with emergency room physicians. Trauma surgeons do surgery and take care of patients throughout the hospital, primarily focusing on the critically ill. Emergency room physicians are certainly front-line workers, but they focus on the initial care of all types of patients, exclusively in the ER. In some countries, orthopedic surgeons deliver trauma care, and anesthesiologists often manage the surgical intensive care units. This is the case in much of Europe. In the United States, general surgeons who have completed medical school (four years), a general surgical residency (five years), and a surgical critical care fellowship (one year) work as trauma surgeons in trauma centers. Some residencies add one or two years of required surgical research. There is no such thing as an official trauma fellowship, as there are no board certifications in trauma. Instead, surgeons take an added board certification in surgical critical care following a fellowship year. As of 2021 in the United States, there were about 3,588 surgeons with board certification in surgical critical care, or about 12 percent of all general surgeons.

The number of board-certified general surgeons in America (about thirty thousand) has been stable for the past thirty years despite a 25 percent increase in the country's population. The limiting factor for producing more surgeons is the small number of surgical residency spots, a number that has changed minimally over the past decades. At the start of the twenty-first century, US medical schools attempted to boost the number of American medical students graduating to increase the physician workforce. This naturally required lowering the criteria for medical school admission. At that time, about 25 percent of surgical residency trainees had attended international medical school programs. They were some of the best and brightest individuals from all over the world. When we increased the number of American medical school positions (by about 25 percent), the postgraduate training space was not changed by growing the size or number of residency spots. We may have replaced some of the brightest surgical residency applicants from international medical schools with folks from US schools because, typically, they get priority even though they may not be as capable, but we have not increased the output of surgeons.

Another concern is that qualified potential applicants to medical school have shied away from a career in medicine due to the enormous cost of education and the length of training. When I attended medical school, my tuition was $400 per year as an in-state resident (at a private school that was in the top ten nationally). Today, at the medical school where I am currently on faculty, the tuition is more than $90,000 per year.

Creating a surgeon certainly requires a long and grueling course of training. During my surgical residency, we were in the hospital every other night and usually awake the entire time. (Think forty hours awake in the hospital and only eight hours at home every forty-eight hours.) My kids, born in the 1990s, say, "Daddy missed the eighties," as I have no recollection of any music produced during that period. The old gray-haired folks from the last generation of surgeons from when I was in training used to say, "The problem with being on every other night is you miss half the action." Meaning that we were missing valuable training experiences if we left the hospital for even a few hours. This was true, but those surgeons lived in the hospital for five years and never left. They had indeed been residents (or occupants) of the facility. Our every other night on call gave us only a tiny, painful glimpse of the real world, which was possibly worse than no glimpse at all.

We used to play a game as interns. Each morning at six o'clock, we asked the medical students to guess who was starting their forty hours on call and who had just finished it. We were all showered and dressed in our little white jackets. The students usually guessed wrong, as the postcall folks were more upbeat and a bit euphoric to be escaping the institution.

> *As a surgeon, one is an optimist—otherwise,*
> *one would not be a surgeon.*
>
> KARL H. BAUER (1890–1978)

The medical community evaluates medical students for personality characteristics, which they use to help predict which field of medicine the trainees are likely to pursue. They are always trying to put individuals into character trait bins. If a student is quiet and cerebral, "internist." If they are eager and energetic, "surgeon." It depends on your perspective. At my medical school, we said, "Surgery is king," as much of the school's leadership and its founder were surgeons. It was generally considered a compliment when you were placed in the "surgeon" box. When I was a medical student, the professors and senior residents often asked me what type of surgeon I would be. I answered that I planned to be a family practitioner like my father. "Nope," they responded every time, "you will be a surgeon." Three days into my surgery rotation, I realized they were correct.

People often say, "Your job must be so stressful." But surgeons tend to be stress resistant. It may be that folks who are calm in the face of a calamity gravitate toward surgery, or it may be that those who survive the grueling residency years can withstand the rigors of a high-intensity career. Indeed, our job is to remain placid when all hell breaks loose. Only by keeping our cool when encountering significant difficulties can we pull patients out of bad situations. More than one chief resident has told me that they were happy that an experienced surgeon was there to calmly deal with a potentially catastrophic problem (usually the audible gushing of blood) encountered during a complex trauma or general surgical procedure. As surgeons, we categorize bleeding as minor, severe, and audible. The latter is when the operative field (essentially the entire abdominal cavity) fills with blood instantaneously when you lighten pressure at the point of bleeding. Typically, this indicates that there is a hole in a large blood vessel. Massive bleeding is dramatic and can be frightening and sphincter-tightening the first few times you see it happen. It is hard to explain to the uninitiated how daunting it can be when bleeding is torrential and the patient's life depends on your getting rapid control. The anxiety provoked can drive many surgical residents (and faculty) to seek other specialty areas within general surgery.

As a senior medical student heading down the path to be a surgeon, I was allowed to place my first chest tube. The chief resident happily guided me through the procedure with a patient on a ventilator in the ICU. It is not particularly scary to do a new procedure with a senior person overseeing you, as they bear all the responsibility. So students and residents generally have little trepidation about doing new things if they are supervised. Alternatively, performing a new procedure as a faculty member, like my first laparoscopic cholecystectomy (removing a diseased gallbladder using tiny incisions aided by television guidance), felt like jumping off a boat into the ocean in the movie The Perfect Storm. *Back to my chest tube. . . . As I inserted the sizeable (~2cm in diameter) plastic tube into the patient's thorax, a massive amount of blood spurted from the thoracic cavity out of the tube and around the hole in the chest wall, splashing onto the bed. I thought I had somehow jammed the tube into the heart. It turned out that this patient needed a chest tube because he was on extremely high ventilator pressure settings, which caused the rapid egress of blood. So I had not caused any damage, but I did become the butt of some surgical humor as an FSA (Future Surgeon of America).*

Some fields of surgery are primarily elective (planned) surgery, involving patients who are not dying (think orthopedics, urology, plastic surgery, or ear, nose, and throat), and some involve more emergency work with patients who are incredibly sick (like much of general surgery, cardiothoracic, neurosurgery, and vascular surgery). All trauma surgeons are general surgeons by training. General surgeons do a wide variety of types of surgery, from which stem a range of surgical specialties, like colorectal, bariatric, breast, surgical oncology, vascular, plastic, and cardiac surgery. (Think of general surgery like the trunk of a large tree, with each surgical specialty representing an important branch.) Trauma surgeons deal with the most death and dying among general surgeons. It is like any other field that attracts a particular kind of person: in this case, the folks who enjoy the challenge of dealing with a patient who is bleeding to death in front of them for unknown reasons gravitate to and remain in the trauma field.

For example, I cringe when I look at the people working high up on bridges or skyscrapers or climbing high mountain peaks, as heights make me shaky. Those who are terrorized by a particular clinical situation focus on other types of practice. The hernia center director who does the same operation under elective conditions multiple times a day is valuable to the community. But the same personality characteristics that make this type of surgeon successful in that endeavor may not be optimal in the uncontrolled environment typically encountered when delivering care to the trauma patient. Without getting dramatic, we trauma surgeons are often called on to act as Captain Sully, landing a jet plane on the Hudson River multiple times every day, sometimes many planes at once.

Trauma surgeons are also called on to help all over the hospital as a ready set of expert hands. So if an obstetrical patient is bleeding during a cesarean section, a trauma surgeon might be called to assist. Or if medical personnel need intravenous access for a patient, they will call on the trauma surgeon. The trauma surgeons, therefore, are the Jack (or Jackie) of all surgical trades, or utility infielders for surgical emergencies. This is not the case for more super-subspecialized surgeons who prefer to "stay in their lane." We try to respond quickly and are there to help deal with every catastrophe.

About fifteen years ago, my colleagues and I did a national survey of trauma centers to assess the supply of trauma surgeons.[1] At that time, the United States had a shortage in the trauma surgeon workforce of about 25 percent. Subsequently, the compensation for trauma surgeons increased, and we have noted more surgeons heading into the field—supply meeting demand.

The knife is dangerous in the hand of the wise,
let alone in the hand of the fool.

HEBREW PROVERB

A little bit of knowledge is a dangerous thing. An individual must mature as a surgical trainee in just a couple of years from checking boxes after

accomplishing tasks as an intern to acting as a full-fledged independent
operator making critical decisions in life-and-death situations. As a
junior resident, I asked my chief residents why a patient had undergone
an operation. "I don't understand the indication for this procedure," I
inquired. "Kids need new shoes" was the typical joking response. But I
did not see the humor in it.

American healthcare carries excessive costs, and surgeons are significant contributors. Recent analysis shows that the US government spends two to three times more per individual per year for healthcare than other developed countries but is significantly behind in critical measures, such as life expectancy, infant mortality, and various quality of life indicators. Why is that? First, doctors' and nurses' yearly incomes have not changed since 1990 (considering inflation), while the cost of healthcare in the United States has skyrocketed. The rise in healthcare spending is related to increases in prices generated by hospitals and insurance companies. For example, while only about 17 percent of Canada's healthcare dollar goes to administration, administration costs represent about 34 percent of the health expenditures in the United States.[2] Our fee-for-service system requires teams of business personnel to fight with each other. So the physician practices have billers fighting with the insurers; the insurers have folks fighting with the doctors and hospitals, and so on. Some people have suggested that the higher costs in the United States are related to research. While we do spend more on research, it is hundreds, not thousands of dollars more per capita. I should mention that I did work for a decade in a state that had very extensive limits on malpractice settlements (favorable tort laws toward physicians). There seemed to be very few malpractice claims. However, I did not observe any differences in physician behavior or defensive medicine practice relative to other states where I have practiced that lack supportive malpractice environments.

Surgeons get paid when they operate in the United States, so there is a real incentive to "cut" in our current fee-for-service environment. For example, let us take a healthy young patient who presents with signs of mild acute appendicitis. In Scandinavia, this person might receive antibiotics. In cases such as this, 80 percent of patients would resolve, and 20 percent would undergo an appendectomy for failure to respond. In the United States, that same patient would likely undergo an appendectomy, as would the majority of such patients. Surgeons are biased because they like to operate—consider the adage "When you are a hammer, the whole world looks like a nail." We are convinced the results are better; we don't focus on the potential complications (surgeons always seem to forget their complications and remember their "saves"); and we, of course, get paid for doing surgery. When surgeons are on flat salaries, the number of borderline indicated (or frankly nonindicated) surgeries diminishes, in my experience. This can backfire, though. In some university practices where everyone is on salary, there is less incentive to do procedures. The "proceduralists" (including surgeons and nonsurgeons who do procedures, like cardiologists, gastroenterologists, and interventional radiologists) may not necessarily be interested in working hard. This all depends on the incentive structure at the institution. I worked at a medical center in Florida where the surgery department had to hire its own surgical endoscopists because the gastroenterologists would not support the surgery service needs. The physician's dedication is certainly more important than whether they have a fixed salaried position or are "killing what they eat" (dependent on their operative volume) or what medical specialty they practice.

Another reason the cost of healthcare in the United States is so high is that a sizable part of the population (some 10 percent, or over thirty million inhabitants) has zero healthcare coverage. Unlike in other developed countries, it is a *privilege* to be healthy rather than a *right* in America. A child in a low-income family with juvenile diabetes does not have the right to the same care as a child born to a family of professionals. But the inequity does not stop there. Studies have shown that the cost of care in the poorest communities in the United States is 400 percent higher than in the rest of the country. When you have no healthcare access, you still receive treatment, usually at safety-net facilities (institutions that provide care regardless of a patient's ability to pay), but the care can be delayed and often more complicated. Rather than prescribing oral antibiotics for an infected mosquito bite on your leg, we must remove a large amount of skin and tissue or amputate your leg because the infection has spread to the surrounding areas.

A few years ago, I was at a surgical conference in Israel where I was asked to participate in a multicenter trial of a new method of treating severe skin and soft tissue infections. I was with my colleague, who ran the trauma center at the Tel Aviv Sourasky Medical Center (a thousand-bed facility), and I asked him why he was not participating. He responded that his facility had only two patients with severe skin infections per year (we had about two per week in the United States at a safety-net hospital less than half the size). In other words, severe skin and soft tissue infections are rare in environments where access to medical care is readily available.

No health coverage (or no care) is superexpensive care that the taxpayers are responsible for covering.

Texas, where I spent part of my career, is at the bottom with Mississippi and Arkansas for the worst healthcare access in the country. Several years ago, I was the on call surgical faculty member responding to general surgical emergencies at both the county hospital and a nearby private hospital. One day I was called by the emergency room of the private hospital about a young woman who was deathly ill, in septic shock from a splenic abscess (pus located in a major blood-filled organ, the spleen). These infections can be quite dangerous. I met the patient and family before surgery and explained the grave situation and the need for surgical intervention. I said we should expect a good result because of the patient's young age but suggested it would have been ideal if she had sought care earlier. They responded that they had spent over a day waiting for care at the county hospital across the street and had carried her to the private hospital ER when she deteriorated.

I was once at a meeting with a young general surgeon in private practice who was advising our department on developing a new bariatric program (surgery on the morbidly obese). I gently asked him why, after six years of surgical training, he wanted to limit his practice to just bariatrics. He reflexively answered that he "could do three cases before noon at about $5,000 each, cash up front." Realizing that this sounded very mercenary, he then added as an afterthought, "and these folks benefit from the procedure." I realized that after almost twenty years in practice at the time, I had no idea how much money was collected on any operation I performed. Trauma surgeons are not concerned with a patient's ability to pay. We just take them as they come.

2

CONTROLLED CHAOS
AT THE TRAUMA CENTER

I dressed him, and God healed him.
AMBROISE PARÉ (1510–1590)

In Paris, France, medical professionals employ a unique prehospital strategy based on the "stay and play" philosophy. This brings trauma resuscitation resources into the street. By contrast, in the United States, this care is provided in the emergency department of a hospital, the "scoop and run" protocol. A notable example of this approach was when Princess Diana was in a horrific car crash in Paris in 1997; she spent more than an hour at the collision scene. When prehospital providers arrived, she was still speaking, but then her heart stopped, and they attempted to revive her in the street. A hospital was only a few miles away. She did have a devastating and complex chest injury, but in North America, we would have tried to move her immediately to a hospital.

Trauma care is delivered in different ways depending on the region. In countries such as Germany, trauma centers are strategically located to serve the geography and population centers and attempt to place everyone within a reasonable distance by helicopter from a receiving hospital. In the United States, such centers seem to be placed in a more random distribution.

In Maryland, for example (with over six million inhabitants), all significant trauma victims are flown to a single adult or solitary pediatric Level I trauma center in Baltimore. The state also has a few Level II trauma centers. (The American College of Surgeons provides a verification process with specific standards of care that the institution must achieve to be declared a Level I [highest level of trauma care] or Level II facility. The primary difference between a Level I and II trauma center is the presence of surgical residents and the quantity of research mandated by this accrediting body.) This is an ideal concentration of resources. In Boston, there are six Level I and one Level II adult trauma centers for a population of under seven hundred thousand in the city proper and 8.5 million in the metro area. Other US states have no grand plan, and there is little statewide governance. I believe that the regionalization of trauma care in fewer, higher-quality centers would lead to better outcomes.

Helicopters are used to transport a patient needing emergent care, and there could be a considerable delay in arriving at a trauma center. The "golden hour" is an artificial invention. Nothing happens at sixty-one minutes postinjury that does not occur at fifty-nine minutes. But military experience with combat casualties has proven that expeditious movement from injury to treatment is optimal. Unfortunately, about 30 percent of Americans are more than an hour away from a trauma center, so their care may be negatively impacted. The mortality rate from car crashes is quite a bit higher per 100 million miles driven in rural areas (like Montana at

1.76 and Wyoming at 1.30) where treatment can be delayed than in states with more urban centers (like New York, 1.02, and New Jersey, 0.88) where collisions may happen much closer to a trauma center.

Just as there are different methods of handling trauma patients throughout various regions in the world, there are also alternative ways to provide care for trauma victims out in the field, like at the scene of a car crash. In the United States, as noted, we "scoop and run" in the prehospital setting. This means we do minimal care for the patient in the street and move them as quickly as possible to the hospital. In years past, interventions such as intravenous infusion of fluids were advocated and sometimes delayed transport. Today, other than placing an airway in a nonbreathing patient or a tourniquet on a bleeding extremity, little intervention is performed at the prehospital setting. Intravenous catheters are usually inserted en route to the facility. In the last decade, blood and blood products, such as plasma, have shown some efficacy particularly for bleeding patients requiring long transport times, like those located in rural areas. About half of trauma deaths are determined at the scene. Of the patients that survive to reach the hospital but succumb to their injuries there, two-thirds bleed to death (usually in the first hour or two), and one-third die from severe brain injury. Fortunately, deaths from trauma total only about 150,000 of the three million injuries per year in the United States, or approximately 5 percent.[1]

The helicopter crew rushed the rancher with a "rattlesnake bite" on his leg to the trauma bay. He had been flown about one hour to the trauma center (about 100 miles). We quickly cut off his clothes but could find no injury. On questioning, this moderately intoxicated middle-aged man denied being bitten by anything. He stated that he had stumbled into his house and told his wife he had seen a rattler, and she had called 911. Fortunately, they had not been watching a documentary on shark attacks . . .

> *How many surgeons does it take to screw in a light bulb?*
> *One—they just hold up the bulb and*
> *the world revolves around them.*
>
> ANONYMOUS

Eric and I had worked on several research projects during his first two years at medical school. During a hiatus to prepare for their board exams, the med students organized a softball game. While running from first base to second, Eric's head collided with the ball. He was knocked unconscious for about half an hour. At the start of the game, Eric was interested in general surgery. After waking up from his head trauma, he changed his intended field to orthopedics. (Clearly, the ball had knocked some sense into him.)

General surgeons and those specializing in trauma are not the easiest people to be around. We tend to be confident, forceful, and commanding, which is a short distance from arrogant, aggressive, and bossy.

Orthopedists tend to be extremely bright, as typically only the top of the class can get into this lucrative field of surgery. And there are few orthopedic residency spots in the United States, so only the best and brightest can compete for these positions. Most of these physicians are friendly and collaborative. While orthopedists are highly competent individuals and could manage all aspects of trauma medical care, in the United States they typically choose to focus just on the bones and joints and leave all other facets of care to the surgical critical care team (the trauma surgeons).

Neurosurgeons can be interesting to deal with. Some years ago, my colleagues and I surveyed neurosurgeons in the United States. Only 8 percent said they specialized in neurosurgical trauma, and many of them wanted to get out of the field. About half of the neurosurgeons in the United States classify themselves as spine surgeons, as that is where the money is. Let's face it, trauma is inconvenient, happening at all hours of the day and night. And it is not lucrative, so it is viewed as a chore. Neurosurgeons can be very rigid about patient management for the injured, as there is little actual research to support what they do in neurotrauma. One hundred percent of the Level I data (the highest level of quality research) in the neurotrauma field are studies that prove that the standard treatment at the time was incorrect. For example, we used to hyperventilate (overbreathe) patients with bad brain injuries and increased brain pressure with the mistaken concept that decreasing brain blood flow would minimize brain swelling. Decades later, this was shown to lead to worse outcomes. Lots of concepts that might seem to be promising ideas turn out to be bad ones. But surgeons, in general, are hard to convince that their dogma may be wrong.

Vascular surgeons are very meticulous and precise and are typically on the cutting edge of medicine. Their field has changed dramatically in the last two decades. They have adopted endovascular surgery (or catheter-based therapy), which is employed with open vascular procedures in most vascular cases today. Part of this operation is performed inside the vessels with catheters under

X-ray control, and part is done with open surgical techniques. In contrast, those individuals specializing in cardiothoracic surgery missed the opportunity years ago to adapt and learn catheter-based therapies. Today, most open cardiac procedures have been replaced with catheter-based procedures, which the medical guys, the cardiologists, perfected. This has left the cardiac surgeons with few procedural morsels left to sustain them.

The challenge of the trauma surgeon is to orchestrate the care of the trauma patient, dealing with all the various surgical personalities and all the medical consultations, and organize the process of care so priorities are met. Each subspecialty appropriately focuses on its particular area, so it is the task of the trauma team to sift through all the recommendations and formulate a safe, efficacious plan of action.

> *He who wishes to be a surgeon should go to war.*
>
> Hippocrates (460–377 BCE)

Much of what we do in trauma care was derived from lifesaving experiences during wartime. A surgeon must always remain adaptable and employ ingenuity to manage demanding situations. In the 1960s, in Vietnam, the "clearing company" was about 50 miles from a facility with an operating room and had few supplies (fluids, a little blood, and a few tubes and surgical instruments) and only young doctors.

A dying soldier with no detectable blood pressure was brought in on a stretcher directly from the battlefield with amputations of his legs and severe injury to his pelvis after an explosion. At that time, hardly any patients with these types of injuries survived. One physician, Bruce Cutler, having completed only two years as a surgical resident before he was deployed, noticed a G-suit that someone had left in the area and got an idea. This anti-gravity apparatus looks like a set of overalls with blood pressure cuffs running up the legs and abdomen. Fighter pilots use it to prevent blood from pooling in the lower extremities during high-G turns, so they do not pass out. Showing initiative, the doc placed the suit on the dying patient, inflated the compartments, and stabilized the patient for transport to higher levels of care. This man survived because of a clever individual's quick thinking and ingenuity. Subsequently, the use of the G-suit was reported in seven more soldiers with devastating injuries in Vietnam, and about half of them lived.

As a resident and junior surgical faculty member in the 1980s, many of the best senior surgeons I worked with had served in Vietnam. One of my grandfathers served with the US Army in the trenches during World War I, and my dad was a navy corpsman in World War II. As someone who did trauma surgery daily, I thought I should join the US Army Reserve to teach trauma. I never anticipated that, eighteen months later, in 1990, US Army Reserve general surgeons would be activated for Operation Desert Storm. I had moved to a new institution just six weeks before to take the position of chief of trauma. The next thing I knew, I was on an air transport jet heading to the Middle East as part of a small, advanced team to help prepare for the arrival of the large field hospital I had been assigned to support. A few weeks later, the entire hospital unit arrived in buses from the airport just as sirens erupted. We were ordered to hit the ground as a Patriot missile rose to strike Scud rockets overhead. The night sky flashed white with the explosion, and missile pieces landed nearby. Shortly after that, our entire hospital unit headed toward Kuwait, where we initially worked to construct a hospital in the desert. I have a great photo of trauma surgeons, orthopedic surgeons, and a gynecologist working as a team, filling sandbags by shoveling sand into a sluice.

Living in the middle of nowhere, there was not much to do most of the time, which is typical of the military experience. One surgeon built a still and started making moonshine. Another developed a technique to create excellent water bagels (he was from Brooklyn). Entertainment was limited, as the entire hospital had few movies to play on the VCR. We probably saw *Pretty Woman* two hundred times. One of the orthopedists and I decided we should have a Passover seder for all the officers during the spring. We somehow got the ingredients to do a complete seder for about forty people, with matzo, chicken soup, and gefilte fish, the whole deal. We even went around the table reading the Passover story.

Before the ground war started, one of the senior surgeons and I helicoptered with some of our most experienced nurses to set up a receiving center for casualties on an airfield in a coastal city. This was challenging because we were told we had forty-eight hours to prepare the newly formed unit to receive thousands of fresh casualties. Fortunately, we only saw about five hundred casualties (mostly Iraqi), and they had been already treated at other facilities. Being a surgeon in a war setting leads to a conflict of interest: we don't like to be idle, but we obviously do not want people to get maimed or killed either.

This experience in Desert Storm led me to become involved with military medicine. First, I developed the Army Trauma Training Center in Miami with Col. Tom Knuth, and later, I trained many military surgical residents and fellows. We created educational opportunities for personnel assigned to visiting forward surgical teams (FST) rotating monthly through the training center. These small units were tasked with stabilizing severely injured military personnel before transport to higher echelons of care. One of the most significant barriers was that the surgical leaders of these teams were accustomed to the peacetime experience, in which all surgery team members were experienced and highly competent and the operative environment was standardized. To instill a sense of the seriousness of the deficit in team dynamics, we constructed operational scenarios that simulated the uncontrolled combat situation. (Many anesthetized pigs died serving their country as part of these experiments, but we felt that our service-people's lives were at stake.) These drills got the attention of the FST unit leaders, who subsequently focused on team training.

I also worked as a consultant for several years at the Institute for Surgical Research, a Department of Defense facility focusing on combat casualty research. Subsequently, I had the opportunity to work with one of my old fellows in Landstuhl, Germany, at the primary receiving hospital for servicepeople returning to the United States after suffering injuries in Iraq and Afghanistan. Incredibly, a soldier could be blown up in the middle of Iraq, managed by the FST, stabilized, and transferred to a larger facility for more definitive work before the nine-hour air transport to Landstuhl. Following a day or two in Germany, these patients traveled to the United States on special transport aircraft with expert personnel and equipment to allow for critical care support the entire trip. A patient who could not breathe independently could be supported on a ventilator or by a special circuit to oxygenate their blood, ECMO, to maintain them on the trip. This enabled victims to survive after incredibly severe injuries sustained in combat.

3

CONSTRUCTING A SURGEON

*The two unforgivable sins of surgery. The first great error
in surgery is to operate unnecessarily; the second,
to undertake an operation for which the surgeon is
not sufficiently skilled technically.*
MAX THOREK (1880–1960)

Medical students go into surgery because they like seeing the
immediate benefits of their intervention. This is in contrast
to the internal medicine service practitioners who often take care
of patients with chronic illnesses, which rarely improve. Both specialties are crucial, but surgeons tend to be more people of action.
My intern "Twin Man"—so named because he and his wife dared
to have twins while he was just an intern—was a perfect example
of this concept.

*Twin Man and I were consulted about an extremely sick man supported
by a ventilator in the medical ICU with a large pleural effusion (free
fluid in the space around the lungs). He looked like he had an infection
with a high fever and elevated heart rate, and we were there to insert a*

large plastic chest tube—the Twin Man's first chest tube. Since I was his supervising resident and responsible for whatever happened, he was naturally gung-ho to do anything. Twin Man prepared the area on the patient's chest wall, made a small incision, and inserted the tube (about 1.5 inches in diameter). Out came a rush of pus. I mean, a lot of pus. It filled the canister, overflowed onto the bed, and seemed to fill the ICU room's floor. The patient was a huge man, and we appeared to have drained multiple liters of pus. He improved before our eyes. To Twin Man, a true individual of action, this was as good as it gets. As we left the ICU, he turned to me and stated bombastically (think Tony the Tiger on the 1970s commercial for Frosted Flakes) the immortal words that we repeated throughout our residency: "Surgery is Grrr . . . EAT." He went on to be one of the foremost plastic surgeons in Florida.

> *You want a surgical team that faces each error, each mishap, straight up, names it, and takes steps to prevent its recurrence.*
>
> FRANCIS D. MOORE (1913–2001)

An intern was "holding the hooks" (a term we use to describe pulling on a large body wall retractor) all night on a complex vascular case performed by a tyrannical vascular surgeon known for devouring residents. The intern started to nod off during the case and awakened while falling backward. He reflexively grabbed the cloth drapes, pulling them off the patient and contaminating the sterile field. He had the good sense to fake a generalized seizure and hit the floor. Everyone felt sorry for him and pulled him out of the operating room to pamper him.

In 1984, a young college student with a history of depression was admitted to a New York hospital. The resident team was in close contact with her family physician. When the patient became agitated, she was prescribed a narcotic that led to a severe drug reaction with one of her depression medications. Her heart stopped, and she died. This drug interaction was virtually unknown by anyone other than a few research scientists. (This was in the days before the internet.) The patient's father was an influential attorney and insisted his daughter had died due to the overwork and lack of supervision of the resident staff. While completely false, his allegations, combined with his political connections, led to the limiting of resident work hours in New York state and, ultimately, nationally. Studies have subsequently shown that resident work hour limitations failed to improve patient outcomes, probably because of a lack of continuity of care, but they have diminished the quality of medical education.[1] In addition, trainee work hour restrictions have elevated medical costs, as someone has to take over all the trainees' workload. Rather than remaining a medical issue, this case became a legal and political matter.

There are misunderstandings about the relationship between hospital work hours and performance. The hospital's hierarchy of clinical decision-making is not related to the fuzzy thinking of a medical student or a tired intern. Most members of the public cannot fathom working more than eighty hours a week. But directing the care of the ill is not the equivalent of working at a desk or a construction site for twenty-four hours straight. When patient care decisions are required, trainees are directed to inform the next-level resident supervisors, and that person discusses the issues with the attending physician. With this tiered approach to patient management, no significant independent decisions are made by junior residents. Unfortunately, rigidly limiting the hours of training has had negative consequences on resident education, particularly in surgery. Many educators feel that trainees in five-year surgery residency programs have lost an entire year (if not more) of experience. This may explain why over 90 percent of surgical residents go on to one- or two-year fellowships after completing their lengthy residencies. They simply do not feel prepared to take on the independent care of the surgical patient when they finish their residency programs.

Imagine you are in your last year of training and are participating in a major operation with a senior surgeon, an operation with which you have limited experience. Because of rigid duty hours limitations, you may be forced to leave in the middle of the case. And because there are many more transitions of care from one resident to another, there are more opportunities for communication breakdown and, therefore, medical errors. There are several so-called index cases that surgical residents must perform before graduation, an experience that continues to be eroded by duty hour restrictions. These index cases are those felt to be essential for trainees to perform, and perform well, prior to being released as competent operators on the public. The data does not support strict eighty-hour duty limitations in surgery residency training programs. Studies have shown that a more flexible work schedule providing a more conducive training environment leads to equivalent care without additional complications or medical errors.

One overlooked issue is that once we surgeons become trauma faculty, we are on call (and responding to general surgical emergencies and trauma cases) and may remain at the hospital, working for twenty-four to thirty-six hours. We often work without sleep but are required to function at the highest level. This is an acquired skill, but it does have negative side effects when returning home after a rough call. My wife refers to me as "post-call Steve": amped up, easily frustrated, and with a hair-trigger temper.

> *Every surgeon carries about him a little cemetery,*
> *in which from time to time he goes to pray,*
> *a cemetery of bitterness and regret, of which he seeks*
> *the reason for certain of his failures.*
>
> RENÉ LERICHE (1879–1955)

The night before the morbidity and mortality conference, in the days before the internet, residents filled the library planning to answer the myriad of possible questions they might be asked if their patient with an adverse event was chosen for discussion. During one memorable conference, a resident was interrogated about why his patient had developed a complication. But this resident had not prepared. After a few faculty members asked him several leading questions without getting a suitable response, the chairman said, "You can just sit down." Every surgery resident in the room became pale and light-headed. This was the worst thing any of us had ever seen at a morbidity and mortality conference. Beatings were routine, and these meetings could be torture for the person presenting a complication, particularly if they were not ready to defend their case. But declaring a resident not even worthy of a thrashing was the ultimate affront.

Most trauma centers hold a weekly morbidity and mortality conference at which selected cases from the previous week's deaths and complications are discussed. This is an essential part of performance improvement and is required for all centers where trauma patients are treated. Each case is presented by a senior surgical resident (usually in their third or fourth year of residency), dissected first by the presenter, and then scrutinized by all faculty members. The faculty member involved must defend the actions leading to complications, as they are responsible for administering the care. The critical features are categorizing the complication or death as preventable, possibly preventable, or nonpreventable and noting what the surgical team could have done differently.

This process is hard to contemplate for the public and even for other practicing physicians, as it can be brutal on both the resident and the staff. When someone does something judged to be incorrect, and that act results in a significant complication or death, the discussion can be harsh. Naturally, the person responsible can experience some guilt or shame, especially if it was a "preventable" error. This can have adverse effects on subsequent clinical performances. But we surgeons must accept responsibility for our actions. Those who perform surgery, particularly trauma surgeons, must undoubtedly learn from their missteps—or, more optimally, from someone else's error. I always paraphrase Albert Einstein that "geniuses learn from other people's mistakes." One of the morbidity and mortality (M and M) conference objectives is for all of us to improve patient care based on the negative experiences of others. It is also an opportunity for wise older surgeons to discuss creative management alternatives that could have prevented a suboptimal outcome. In some instances, everything may have been done according to the standard of care, but the patient had a bad outcome anyway. In these circumstances, we may inquire about what we could do differently next time. I have a desk plaque one of my surgical research fellows gave me before she left to complete her surgical training: "There is NO crying in Surgery." (I should note that there are some excellent books analyzing the morbidity and mortality conference process, including *Forgive and Remember* by Charles Bosk.)

Surgeons must dispassionately learn from judgment errors. Ultimately, however, we need a tiny rearview mirror so that when the next emergency arises, one that requires rapid decision-making, we won't be paralyzed by the fear of making another error. The best lay comparison is an NFL quarterback afraid to throw a tough pass because the last attempt was intercepted. For a surgeon, failure to make immediate (and correct) decisions can cost lives. We can't carry the weight of every poor outcome, bad trauma, or critically ill patient; if we did, we wouldn't be able to care for the next patient. Or the next.

> *All truth passes through three stages:*
> *First, it is ridiculed. Second, it is violently opposed.*
> *Third, it is accepted as being self-evident.*
>
> ARTHUR SCHOPENHAUER (1788–1860)

When I was a senior medical student on "professor" rounds (a weekly teaching exercise) with the resident team, we had a patient who had sustained an abdominal gunshot wound to a major vessel (inferior vena cava), and his legs were wrapped to the groin with ACE bandages in an attempt to prevent venous pooling and subsequent thrombosis of veins. I had read that an anticoagulant (Heparin) was routinely being used at other institutions to prevent venous clot formation. I inquired with the faculty member (a very senior surgeon who was the chief of surgery at this large county hospital) about using Heparin on our high-risk patient. The professor looked at the chief resident and asked, "Where do they get this stuff?" and laughed.

In medical school, there was a strong surgical service dogma regarding all forms of patient management. And heaven help you if you diverged from institutional protocol and a patient did not do well. I moved to the Northeast for my residency and soon after was asked by my surgery chairman, "What's the data?" I had never heard this question uttered by a surgeon while in medical school. I became convinced that understanding the evidence supporting our care was essential long before it was called "evidence-based medicine" (EBM). It turns out that Scottish surgeon John Hunter urged his pupils to understand the scientific basis for medical care as early as the 1700s. Unfortunately, only about 25 percent of the care we give in medicine today is supported by high-level quality science, so much of what we do is based on clinical experience. But when there is data that supports a particular patient care method, most doctors feel we should use it. And when there is not, we need to investigate that issue and generate quality information to direct our treatment. One problem is the massive quantity of data that inundates us every month. Surgeons need someone to take the time to sift through the relevant material on each topic, digest it, and tell us the best care for each situation. I have edited a few textbooks focusing on EBM in surgery to meet some of those needs.[2]

But where does this data come from? The answer is research, but, more specifically, "translational" research. This is scientific evidence based on a clinical issue ("bedside"), which is studied either in the laboratory or through a rigorous clinical trial ("bench"), and then returned to the "bedside" to be applied to patient care. For example, in the 1990s, there was a rash of horrible liver injuries after car crashes. Many seat belts were configured in two pieces at the time, and riders often wore only the automatic shoulder part and did not lock the lap belt portion. In major collisions, the shoulder harness cut into the abdomen and sort of guillotined off the back of the liver. Further exacerbating the problem was that the regimen for resuscitating hemorrhaging trauma patients involved massive volumes of fluids. All that fluid diluted clotting factors, which in some instances led to the development of a significant coagulopathy (inability to clot). So the combination of a complex liver injury and poor clotting of blood ended in death by hemorrhage in some of our trauma patients. Some of my colleagues participated in the Crash Injury Research and Engineering Network (CIREN), a federally funded consortium of trauma centers dedicated to better understanding vehicular injury and identifying the causative issues. Subsequently, car manufacturers made some significant seat belt design changes. In addition, the substantial number of patients bleeding to death from the liver led our group and others to develop new animal models of liver injury. We were able to identify some novel bandages and clotting aids to facilitate bleeding control. These techniques were then brought back to the bedside (the operating room), which helped save lives.

So much of what we do in medicine is based on attributing importance to something we can measure or observe (regardless of whether it is vital) just because we were told to do so in training. Unfortunately, as stated above, we have quality data to create evidence-based patient management protocols in only a small percentage of circumstances. Therefore, we use the "art" of medicine to guide our care in most situations. And it can be challenging, if one is not rigorous, to differentiate the art from the science guiding patient management.

You snooze; you lose.

From a 1968 TV commercial for
a mattress store in Oshkosh

The chief resident had been dawdling as he completed an appendectomy when he got a call that a trauma patient was on the way. Surgical residents love to operate, so they sometimes try to stretch out the case a little bit. As the trauma surgeon attending on call, I scrubbed out of the case (I removed my gloves and sterile gown over my scrub suit) as the resident was finishing and headed down to meet the patient. When I arrived at the ER, we were notified that the patient had a stab wound to the left chest. As a precaution, we removed the chest tray from its sterile wrapper and prepared all the instruments in case a thoracotomy (opening the chest) was required. This preparation for a major chest procedure is performed often, but we rarely need to do this intervention. We commonly place a chest tube to decompress air or blood in the chest cavity (for pneumothorax or hemothorax). Only patients dying in front of us from chest wounds warrant a thoracotomy.

I was with a second-year surgical resident as the patient rolled through the door. This young stab wound victim with a hole in his left chest had conversed while in the ambulance but had lost vital signs as he entered the trauma room. I guided the ecstatic junior resident through his first emergency thoracotomy. This rare, life-saving procedure is always stolen from the junior residents by those more senior. I guess they all want the chance to be a hero. After placing a Finochietto retractor, the resident opened the pericardial sac around the heart, and a gush of blood came

out. The heart started to beat again. I helped the junior resident place a
finger over a hole in the heart and use a stapler to close the defect. The
stapler is preferred over sutures, as surgeons often stab themselves with the
needle when repairing the beating heart. (Remember, the heart is pound-
ing, and a surgeon's hand bounces with each beat. It is easy to skewer your
hand with a needle.) We then placed a towel over the chest cavity and
readied the patient to head to the OR for formal repair of the heart and
closing of the chest wall. As a senior surgeon, I had done many of these
cases and had quite a few successes. Just as I do not get very down with
trauma tragedy, I do not get excited about a significant victory. The
junior resident, however, was jumping for joy. Just then, the chief resi-
dent showed up. "What's happening?" he asked us. "We just cracked his
chest, fixed his heart, and he is doing fine," I responded. The chief resi-
dent's face fell. He had missed an opportunity to have a major "save." As
they say, "You snooze, you lose."

Many thoracotomies are performed for traumatic cardiac arrests,
but they are rarely lifesaving procedures. Years ago, we looked at
the national success rate if a patient arrived at the hospital without
a heartbeat or detectable blood pressure after trauma, and we
found that only about 2 percent survived. The results are much
better when someone arrives alive and dies in front of you.

> *The interns suffer not only from inexperience*
> *but also from over experience.*
>
> WILLIAM STEWART HALSTED (1852–1922)

His friends took away his car keys, dragged him intoxicated from the bar
to his home, and put him in bed. When the patient awoke, he jumped on

his motorcycle and crashed into a tree, breaking his back and severing his spinal cord. He was found paralyzed at the scene by the paramedics. Now permanently paraplegic, he sued the bar, his friends, me, the trauma surgeon, and my hospital. Why sue me?

This injury occurred during the first week of July (the week the new academic year starts). On her first night of call, a new surgical intern wrote in the medical record that the patient was "moving all four extremities" (which is the default "normal" neurological exam). During my deposition, the plaintiff's attorney asked me what we had done to the patient to cause his paraplegia, as he was "moving" in the emergency room but was paralyzed when he arrived at the ICU. I responded that we did nothing, but the intern had written an erroneous statement. I displayed the spine surgeon's operative note describing the absence of the spinal cord for many inches. Nothing we did could have caused that. They immediately dropped the case.

On the first of July every year, a new set of doctors start their residency. On that day, every level of residency moves up a year, assuming the duties of the next-higher rank. Senior medical students become interns, and so on. Imagine that all the privates in the army became sergeants on a particular day, and all the lieutenants became captains, and so on, without necessarily earning the advancement. The first two years of surgical residency are considered the junior years, during which the trainees are given little responsibility. The big advancement hurdle occurs when surgical residents move into the third year of residency. Senior residents are considered highly responsible and informed in the third year and above. They are expected to make correct decisions every time or at least recognize when they cannot. Because everyone matures at different rates during training, it can be tough to determine who will make a good surgeon. A lot of faculty time and discussion are expended in the promotion process, but that process can backfire. I recently worked in a residency program with a fine gentleman who was going through surgical training at the same age as most of the faculty. He had a fantastic attitude, and everyone agreed he was a wonderful human being. He was certainly dedicated to providing optimal care to his patients. Unfortunately, he just did not have enough horsepower to quickly and efficiently manage the surgical workload and make rapid decisions. And he was not technically proficient. He repeated his second year and did three third years before he was finally dropped from the program. This was best for both the resident and the program, but they should have made this decision years previously.

This brings up the phenomenon I call the "second-slowest antelope." It is sometimes stated that folks in Arkansas love the state of Mississippi because, if not for Mississippi, Arkansas would be considered the all-around worst state in the United States. The second-slowest antelope concept pertains to the people who are doing a marginal job as surgical residents but are completely ignored because there is someone in the program that is much worse and is the focus of everyone's attention. The gentleman mentioned above, whom the faculty was agonizing over how to help improve, was just such an individual. That is why rigorous criteria for promotion in surgery are essential. Having underperformers can bring down the quality of the entire surgical residency program.

I should mention that the technical ability to operate is rarely a factor in advancement. Maybe 2 to 3 percent of surgeons are genuinely gifted, skilled technical geniuses (think Denton Cooley, who was one of the world's most famous cardiovascular surgeons). These rare surgeons can operate like nobody else, whereas a small percentage of individuals simply cannot use their hands (they somehow lack the dexterity required to do even the most basic of operations). In between these two groups, about 95 percent of surgeons are technically competent. The decision about whom to operate on and when to do it and how to manage the patient is what separates the best surgeons from those who are not as talented. Rarely is it technical brilliance that differentiates surgeons.

When I finished training, I joined a brilliant surgeon-scientist, Dr. F, an excellent critical care doctor and a capable surgeon (he went on to become a chairman of surgery at one of the prestigious Harvard hospital programs). He told me about the day he went to see his program director to quit his surgical residency and change to primary care. He was in a navy surgical training program during the Vietnam War era. Dr. F was very well regarded as a surgical resident by the faculty and was thought to be doing an excellent job. Why would he want to leave the residency? Dr. F related that he operated on straightforward inguinal hernias a couple of days per week with another junior resident, whom we will call Dr. Burke. In each case, they would alternate who would be the surgeon versus the assistant. "Every day, I operate with Burke. It takes me thirty to forty minutes to complete hernia repairs. But Burke can do them all in five or ten minutes," said Dr. F. He concluded, "I just can't operate like Burke." The program director, a senior surgeon, responded, "Hey, I can't operate like Burke." It turns out that Dr. Burke was one of those rare technically gifted individuals. He went on to be one of Denton Cooley's cardiothoracic surgical fellows.

Once you start studying medicine,
you never get through with it.

CHARLES H. MAYO (1865–1939)

One of my old professors used to say, if a medical student wants to use
ketchup as a blood substitute, don't laugh at them. They may go on to
discover the next oxygen-carrying fluid. So educators must be welcoming
to all interested individuals. For example, Javier wanted to work in our
animal research laboratory. He had completed university in the United
States but returned to his native Colombia for medical school, likely
because of the cost savings of schooling at home. The cost of medical school
education in America is astronomical. (As of 2022, the average US stu-
dent has a debt of more than $150,000 when they graduate, and about
half owe more than $200,000.) My attitude is that any student or resi-
dent that expresses a research interest is welcome. Only a tiny fraction of
those who do express an interest follows through, however. Javier was one
of those who followed through. He started volunteering every day in the
lab and soon ran many of the experiments. We started paying him a full
salary as a research technician. Then Javier began to help design projects
that were published under his name. We arranged a scholarship for him
to obtain a master of public health. On completing his thesis, he found an
excellent surgical residency spot and then a great fellowship. Later, Javier
became a surgical faculty member at a prestigious university and obtained
a National Institutes of Health grant.

Only about 10 percent of surgeons in the United States are academic surgeons, which means 90 percent are in private practice or
primarily clinical care. Academic surgeons usually have research
focus areas and are expected to be surgical educators, training

medical students and surgical residents. Private practice surgeons are often actively involved in teaching. Due to time constraints and the need to generate income from their clinical practice, they rarely have significant involvement in research. Most surgical education in hospitals occurs in the operating room. Because operating room time is not predictable, the trauma and surgical intensive care surgeons also spend a considerable amount of time teaching residents and students during patient care rounds at the bedside. In addition, there is a plethora of conferences every day at which patient care is discussed in considerable detail. For example, we conduct a daily "morning report" meeting, during which all the admissions from the previous day are reviewed, along with any issues concerning complicated patients on the service. This provides an essential level of oversight and adds a layer of checks and balances.

Incidentally, hospitals with surgical residents have been shown to have better patient outcomes, even though operations take a little bit longer with a resident performing part or all of the case, depending on their level of training and capabilities. I love collaborating with residents and have done so for my entire career. While at times frustrating, being able to help an individual develop into a fully formed, competent surgeon is something I find very gratifying. As a person who truly hated school and had some terrible teachers, I dedicated myself long ago to trying to emulate the outstanding educators I did encounter. I found during my residency that learning educational material at the level required to instruct another person forced me to have a much better grasp of the subject.

I also learned how *not* to do things during my years in training and afterward. For example, I once worked with a chief of surgery at the city hospital who would play favorites. If he favored you, he would speak to you. If not, he would lay in wait, ready to pounce on any misstep. When I was a chief resident, one of my fourth-year residents was so intimidated from fear of being attacked by this faculty member for making the wrong decision that he could not make any decisions. In contrast, one of my all-time favorite professors, Dr. Hoye, used to intentionally release retractors or remove clamps during procedures to force the residents to learn to operate independently (while never putting the patients at risk, I should add). This, while quizzing the operating resident about every aspect of the physiology and anatomy of the operation. One faculty member reminisced about the time he appeared in the operating room as a resident, utterly unprepared for one of Dr. Hoye's operations. He said it was the longest three hours of his life. When Dr. Hoye retired, all the residents got together and bought him a huge antique German nutcracker in remembrance of his unique and wonderful teaching style. He was amazing. Having high expectations and being tough on the surgical trainees while supporting their development, as was the case with Dr. Hoye, is highly desirable. The abuse and favoritism by the chief of surgery mentioned above, however, were demoralizing and more in the realm of harassment by a bully.

What's the most conservative thing to do?
STEPHEN M. COHN, M.D.

The little boy was flown to the trauma center with his siblings and his parents who were injured when their "coyote's" van, which was smuggling them across the border, ran off the road and flipped over. Immigration and the local vigilantes were in pursuit when they crashed. The entire family was severely injured, but the six-year-old was in the worst shape. He was in a state of shock and could not move his legs. He had sustained significant injuries to his abdominal aorta (the primary blood vessel supplying his abdomen and legs) and intestines, and his lumbar spine and spinal cord had been crushed. We repaired his aorta and other abdominal injuries and got him through a difficult postoperative course. For weeks, he was paralyzed and could not move his legs. Miraculously, he later regained the use of his legs and was able to walk again.

Trauma surgeons are often asked how we deal with the disasters we see on the job. We tend to not dwell on past cases to an excessive degree. We accept tragic outcomes as something we cannot alter outside of population-based injury prevention programs. It can be frustrating when a societal solution is not adopted, like banning assault rifles, which seemed like an obvious choice after the Sandy Hook Elementary School and, more recently, the Robb Elementary School massacres. My children were at the midnight premiere of the Batman movie *The Dark Knight Rises* in July 2012 when a young man in a Colorado theater opened fire, killing twelve and injuring fifty-nine. My children were in a theater in another state, but I remember thinking it could have been them.

I look at my patients' loss-of-life issues in a detached way, particularly when the patients are adults. I understand the systematic way that we must evaluate the trauma victim. If we follow well-established management protocols, then we do not feel responsible for bad patient outcomes. I always try to do the most conservative thing at every decision point. Those who are well-trained and have common sense and good judgment certainly try to avoid errors.

Therefore, surgeons must be careful observers. During residency training, we see methods of surgical care that work and those that do not. There is a saying that I abhor, which we use when someone does everything wrong but "gets away with it." We say, "Better lucky than good." As residents and in our surgery practice, we learn the most conservative (or safest) approach and see examples of how diverging from this process can lead to catastrophe. While there may be multiple correct paths, the most conservative approach is always my preference. This philosophy is employed in situations where there is no clear path forward and no experience with a particular unique circumstance. My wise former chief resident used to say, "There are five hundred ways of doing everything in medicine, and two hundred and fifty are correct. Pick one of them." In trauma and surgery, I strive to always stay within the established parameters of safe care. This does not prevent me from saying at our morbidity and mortality conference, "So we did everything according to the standard of care, but the patient died. What can we do differently moving forward?" This does not suggest the surgical team did anything wrong but rather that we need to rethink the issue and investigate the problem. That can be the nidus for research that leads to significant advancements that occur in patient management.

Thus, when we do everything according to the best practice, I do not feel responsible when an adult patient dies. I might feel sad, but I do not wallow in those emotions. We often have multiple other patient responsibilities to oversee simultaneously, which can make excessive reflection detrimental to the care of the next patient. However, I do feel bad for children who die because they are so vulnerable. It is sometimes the case that adults put them in harm's way, like when a small child is killed while playing with a loaded handgun left lying around the house. They remind me so much of my own kids that I can empathize. When a child dies, we always feel awful. But we do not have the luxury of mourning for too long, as the next traumas are already rolling in the trauma center door.

Medical students must start this process of compartmentalization early. On our first surgery rotation, a group of fellow students and I were assigned to cover the ER at the bustling county hospital where every few nights we were deluged with the consequences of violence. There was a small "sewing" room in the back of the ER where the medical students were tasked with closing the lacerations of a continuous stream of patients. In addition, we were expected to respond to all the codes that occurred. A loud bell would sound to notify everyone of a medical cardiac arrest, and a buzzer went off when there was a trauma code. This went on seemingly continuously, night and day. There was even a glass-walled room the size of a phone booth from which freshman medical students could observe all the goings-on. They were required to wear white scrubs so no one would ask them to do anything, and they were squeezed in tightly with their fresh faces pushed up against the glass. One morning at about two o'clock, another hungry, dog-tired student and I were headed to the cafeteria when we were stopped by two dudes dragging an unresponsive man by the armpits, a bloody splotch blossoming on his chest. He was hemorrhaging from a gunshot wound. "Where is the emergency room?" they yelled. We thumbed in the direction behind us, not even turning our heads or moving to help. Moments later, we heard the buzzer ring.

A few months before writing this book, I experienced a very sad situation. Rather than box up my feelings and place them somewhere in the recesses of my mind, I had to tell my wife this story when I came home one night. A baby girl, maybe eight months old, had sustained a terrible brain injury when she was brutally abused by a parent. The actual events of the injury were murky, as they often are. The story was that the child had fallen down some stairs, but of course, babies this young cannot walk and typically are not mobile enough to fall down a flight of stairs. But this child was dying of severe brain damage and lying in a tiny crib on a ventilator in a large room in the pediatric ICU, all alone. Normally, children in the PICU are surrounded by anxious family members hovering at the bedside, watching their every breath. But the family was barred from the bedside by child protective services while an investigation was ongoing. I remember thinking how dreary, stark, and lonely it was in the big, empty room filled only with the sound of the ventilator triggering as it breathed for the dying baby. You just never see a baby alone in the hospital like this. Somehow, the imminent demise of an innocent child from devasting brain injury in complete isolation made the situation even more tragic and moving than usual. So while we can compartmentalize in most situations, some tragedies strike us to our core.

4

GENERALIST SURGEONS

My work essentially has been that of plumber of the alimentary canal. I have worked on both ends, but largely in between.
Owen H. Wangensteen (1898–1981)

A middle-aged woman presented with projectile vomiting, abdominal distention, and clinical and radiological signs of bowel obstruction (gastrointestinal tract blockage). She was taken to the operating room by one of my surgical partners for abdominal exploration. Her stomach and small intestine were massively dilated and filled with sizeable chunks of unchewed pineapple. An enormous number of these fruit pieces were removed from her stomach—enough to fill a large bucket. The patient was in septic shock and multiorgan failure for a few days. When she finally recovered, everyone wanted to know how this had happened. It turns out that a friend came back from a trip to Mexico with a large bag of freeze-dried pineapple pieces, and she consumed them all in one sitting. No doubt she followed her pineapple gluttony with some form of liquid beverage . . .

Most operative procedures on our trauma patients involve repairing broken bones, which is performed by orthopedic surgeons. There is little operatively for general/trauma surgeons to perform in the trauma population, as few patients need abdominal or chest surgery after injury. In the 1980s, before the widespread availability of the computed tomography (CT) scanner, there were many more operations for trauma. For example, an injury to the spleen (the large blood-filled organ in the upper-left abdomen) led to an operation more than 85 percent of the time in 1989 but only about 25 percent of the time in 2010. Surgery to remove the spleen related to trauma, performed weekly just a few years ago, is now required only a few times per year at most trauma centers. It was not recognized before then that most of these injuries could be observed and would cease bleeding and heal without removal of the spleen. Today, we successfully treat most abdominal and chest trauma without operative intervention. Except for inner-city trauma centers where there is more penetrating violence, such as gunshot wounds or stab wounds (these patients have a much higher likelihood of needing an operation), today's general surgeons typically do not see many trauma patients necessitating operative intervention.

In addition to delivering all the nonoperative care to trauma patients, trauma surgeons provide critical care services. Usually, they function as surgical hospitalists, aiding providers throughout the hospital. With little trauma to operate on, we instead perform most emergency general surgery cases at hospitals with a trauma center. This includes managing acute appendicitis and inflamed gallbladders and taking care of almost anything that is perforated, obstructed, or bleeding.

So I might have the immense privilege of relieving
the pain, anguish, and threat to a wonderful small boy
by making an incision in the right lower quadrant of his
abdomen and taking out a pus-filled appendix skillfully
and safely, my first operation. I felt that this was both
a miracle and a privilege. I still do.

FRANCIS D. MOORE (1913–2001)

We took a seventeen-year-old woman with appendicitis to the operating room. Once she was under anesthesia, we palpated a lump in the right lower quadrant of the abdomen because she was very thin. We made a small incision (5 millimeters) over this area. On entering the peritoneal cavity, out popped "the worm," the inflamed appendix. After placing clamps, we removed the appendix and put one stitch in the fascia, one suture under the skin, and one of those little round Band-Aids over the wound. In the morning, the patient was amazed that we had performed an entire operation through such a tiny incision.

The presence of the appendix was unknown until the fifteenth century because much of our knowledge of human anatomy for about twelve centuries was based on the anatomic studies of Galen. Galen studied monkeys, who lack an appendix. The appendix exists in humans, rabbits, and some primates and marsupials, but it is otherwise rare across animal species. No one knows the purpose of this structure. It is possible that the appendix—a small outpouching from the first part of the large intestine—represents a safe house from which gut bacteria could repopulate the rest of the intestine after a catastrophic illness, like earthlings returning from a Martian colony after the home planet was devastated.

In the 1300s, English barber surgeons (barbers with no formal university training who performed primitive operations) mentioned inflammation in the lower right of the abdomen, the first suggestion of appendicitis. One of the first graphic depictions of the appendix was produced in 1492 by Leonardo da Vinci. It was not until the eighteenth century that appendicitis with perforation (when the appendix bursts) was first reported. Around that time, John Hunter, the first surgeon-scientist, initially described the gangrenous appendix. Amazingly, operations occurred in the 1700s to remove these appendixes without anesthesia, but these had little success and often ended in death. It was not until 1880 that the first successful appendectomy was performed in England. In 1886, Reginald Fitz, an American pathologist, attributed this inflammatory condition to the appendix and was the first to coin the term "appendicitis." As a result, appendectomies became commonplace but were still associated with significant mortality before antibiotics.

About 10 percent of Americans are diagnosed with acute appendicitis during their lifetime. This is usually a disease of the young, with a median age of twenty-two, and is found most commonly in the second decade of life, but it can occur at any age. About 325,000 appendectomies are completed in the United States each year, making it one of the more common operations. Appendicitis can be hard to diagnose, as only 25 percent of the time do patients with appendicitis present with the classic signs and symptoms of the disease. This is because the appendix hides in the back of the abdomen about 80 percent of the time and therefore may not show the usual signs of disease until late and the inflammatory process is quite advanced. It is not surprising that in about 22 percent of patients, the appendix has perforated by the time they arrive at the hospital ER. Perforation, unfortunately, increases the risk of infectious complications by about ten times.

Many famous people have died from acute appendicitis. A partial list includes Brigham Young, who started the Mormon Church; escape artist Harry Houdini; and, more recently, political leader Daniel Patrick Moynihan. And many well-known people have survived appendicitis and gone on to successful careers: artist Henri Matisse (see below), the founder of neurosurgery Harvey Cushing, tennis star Suzanne Lenglen, General Dwight D. Eisenhower, President Gerald Ford, musician Elton John, and many more.

There is an interesting tale about Henri Matisse, who, as a young man, developed complicated acute appendicitis in the days before antibiotics. He was a law student and had to convalesce at home on bed rest for an extended period. The story goes that Matisse's mother bought him some art supplies to relieve him of boredom. Much to his father's dismay, Henri gave up the study of law and decided to become an artist. And the rest is history . . .

*In the future, everyone will be
world-famous for fifteen minutes.*

ANDY WARHOL, WHO DIED FROM A CARDIAC ARRHYTHMIA
WHILE RECOVERING FROM GALLBLADDER SURGERY (1928–1987)

We were called to see a dying woman in her forties in the medical intensive care unit. No one understood why she was so extremely sick. Overnight, this otherwise healthy woman had developed failure of essentially all of her organs. She was having convulsions, she was on maximum support from the ventilator, she was receiving three drugs at a maximum

*dose to support her heart, her kidneys were not working, her liver had
failed (her bilirubin—the pigment formed in the liver and excreted in
the bile—was 50; normal is around 1), and even her bone marrow had
shut down. She was too sick to move to get any imaging, so her ICU team
ordered a bedside ultrasound as a last-ditch effort to find something,
anything that could be corrected. Her gallbladder looked exceptionally
large but had no stones. It was impossible to interpret any other findings.*

*Usually, we would avoid operating on a moribund patient, but she
was so young that we decided to intervene with the hope of finding a
reversible problem. She barely survived the trip to the operating room.
On abdominal exploration, we found an enormous black, dead gallbladder. We quickly removed the diseased organ. Immediately, on the operating table, she started to improve. In medical school in the South, we
heard the old adage, "Piss and pus must pass." It means we need to take
out all the obstructed body fluids and diseased organs. Removing the
source of infection or a dead structure (like this gangrenous gallbladder)
can rapidly improve overall status. This was one of the few cases that I put
in the "near miracle" category, as within twenty-four hours of surgery,
her lungs were returning to normal, her heart was pumping at baseline,
and her kidneys and liver were normalizing. A week later, she went
home. We rarely see patients getting this ill from gallbladder disease, and
she was one of the sickest people I have ever seen who survived.*

It seems like the world's population is just chock-full of gallstones
(really, about 20 percent of Westerners and 10 percent of Asians
develop this condition). These stones form in supersaturated bile
from the body's biochemical compounds such as cholesterol, bile
salts, and lecithin. The likelihood of making gallstones is related
to gender (two-thirds are in women) and racial makeup, but it is

not genetic (meaning, it is not inherited like, for example, hemo-philia, which parents pass to their children through a gene on the X chromosome). The highest prevalence of stones appears to be in Native Americans and the Hispanic population of Central and South America. This is likely not related to diet, but fatty foods do stimulate the gallbladder to contract and can precipitate a gall-bladder attack, during which a stone lodges in the outflow tract of bile from the gallbladder, causing pain. Fortunately, only about 20 percent of folks with gallstones ever have symptoms, so many peo-ple are walking around with little rocks in their gallbladders.[1] But among people who develop symptoms (typically a dull pain in the upper-right abdominal region after a fatty meal), more than half of them will have another episode within a year. These second episodes can be more problematic and long-lasting with a more complicated disease course, so we try to remove the culprit after the first episode of symptoms.

The gallbladder (like the appendix) does not seem to have much of a purpose, as evidenced by the fact that there appear to be no consequences of not having one. Extensive studies have looked at everything from bowel function to cancer and found zero impact of the lack of a gallbladder. This is a good thing because removing the gallbladder is among the most common operations performed worldwide, with over 700,000 each year in the United States alone. In the days before laparoscopy (where we make small incisions and operate while using a camera), this procedure (cholecystectomy) was performed open via an incision under the right rib cage. This was a safe procedure but was associated with considerable pain and some respiratory compromise in the postoperative period. Today, most gallbladders are removed laparoscopically. The process is more difficult technically for the surgeon, but there is much less postoperative discomfort for the patient. Currently, patients have short hospital stays (usually less than twenty-four hours) compared to three to five days in the "old" days. From the surgical educator's perspective, doing this procedure laparoscopically converted an enjoyable operation that was often performed by a junior resident into a more difficult one, often with a higher-level resident. The operative strategy for accomplishing this procedure safely has not changed, but the technique employed makes assessing the anatomy much more difficult. The surgeon must visualize the bile ducts, gallbladder, and liver adequately and correctly identify each structure. The problem lies in the fact that, unlike in a textbook, there are no labels on the structures. More concerning is the variability of the biliary anatomy (only 25 percent of people have a "normal" anatomic layout). Also, the ducts can be very tiny in smaller people, particularly women, adding another complexity level. The final concept that is important to understand is that if a bile duct is injured, it is a surgical catastrophe necessitating major ductal reconstruction. While rare (occurring in about one in four thousand cholecystectomies), bile duct injuries are a known complication, occurring even in the most experienced hands.

> *No disease of the human body, belonging to the province*
> *of the surgeon, requires in its treatment, a better combination*
> *of accurate anatomical knowledge with surgical*
> *skill than a hernia in all its varieties.*
>
> Astley Paston Cooper (1768–1841)

We planned to repair a massive chronic inguinal hernia (a hernia is a weak spot or other abnormal opening in a body wall that can permit tissue or parts of an organ to bulge through). The scrotum of this morbidly obese man was filled with a giant hernia containing much of his large intestine. This hernia was hanging down to his knees and causing symptoms of intermittent intestinal blockage. At the start of the case, we could not locate the man's penis, so we called the urology service to help. They were also unsuccessful in finding his penis. We explored his groin, only to find much of his colon in his scrotum. We resected the colon and repaired the hernia floor with mesh. At the end of the operation, having removed a basketball-sized volume of tissue, we (and the urologists) again failed to find the penis. One wonders how this man urinated before arriving at the hospital.

Inguinal hernias (bulges in the groin area) develop in about 25 percent of all men (and only 2 percent of women). Men are particularly prone to developing an inguinal hernia due to the way testicles descend during development through a space called the processus vaginalis. This space is supposed to close in the few weeks before and after birth. Most inguinal hernias, therefore, are seen in men, and fortunately, most men have them dealt with long before their penis disappears. There was a time when, if we found an asymptomatic hernia, we would operate on it to repair this weakness in the tissues. We did this to avoid enlargement of the hernia over time or the dreaded complication of tissue or an organ becoming stuck in this defect. We no longer take this approach because many hernias do not require repair. Waiting for patients to develop hernia-related symptoms in most cases precludes unnecessary operations.

Some of the most common hernias that surgeons deal with are ventral and incisional hernias. These can occur naturally (umbilical hernias at the navel) or after major abdominal surgeries, when they manifest as a defect at the incision site. Repairing these hernias can be problematic, particularly for the obese. We fix both incisional and inguinal hernias with a plastic mesh because avoiding tension during the repair is essential to its success. Even surgery on tiny umbilical hernias (bulges in the belly button) is ten times more successful when a mesh is used instead of performing a primary repair with sutures. So if you undergo a hernia repair today, you will typically receive a piece of mesh to help bridge the gap in the tissues and avoid excessive stress. Fortunately, the mesh is inert and sterile and rarely contributes to any complications of these repairs.

No drainage is better than the ignorant employment of it.

WILLIAM STEWART HALSTED (1852–1922)

"He pulled out his NG tube again without using his hands," claimed the senior ICU nurse. "Come on," I said, incredulously, "this is like the fourth time this guy has pulled his NG tube out." (NGs, or nasogastric tubes, suck the air out of the stomach. They are commonly used in patients on ventilators, who swallow a lot of air.) She responded, "I have him in full restraints, and he just spits out the tube." We stopped our clinical care rounds and replaced the stiff plastic tube through this wide-awake patient's nose and down into his stomach and secured it in place. Then, before our eyes and in full four-extremity restraints, he pushed the tube out of his nose onto the bed. He used only his talented tongue, which was quite facile. No one had ever seen this before or since.

In the 1930s, a famous surgical leader suggested that nasogastric (NG) suction-siphonage (his term) would be beneficial after abdominal operations. The surgical world accepted this suggestion with no comparative data as if it had been handed down from Moses. For over fifty years, it remained dogma. More patients complained about the discomfort from the NG tube in their nose than about the huge incision in their abdomen. And there were entire medieval rituals around NG removal. Some surgeons wanted the tube clamped for hours before removal. Others required their patients to have a bowel movement as evidence of the return of gut function. Both measures prolong the agony of having an unnecessary NG tube. These patients were so miserable from the irritation of the tube that they took a lot of painkillers (such as narcotics) to be more comfortable, which further slowed the return of peristalsis. In the days of widespread NG use, patients often spent a week in the hospital and required a tube for two to three days after a routine, uncomplicated open appendectomy. Today, after a typical appendectomy performed open or laparoscopic, the patient leaves the same or next day, without ever needing an NG tube.

In the mid-1980s, several clinical trials demonstrated that the NG tube did nothing to prevent postoperative complications in intestinal surgery. When I was a senior surgical resident rotating on a busy colorectal service, the word came down to stop using NG tubes in elective colon cases. The service changed overnight as previously miserable patients transformed into happy-faced individuals wondering when they could eat and go home.

The wound should be treated in such a way as to produce suppuration as quickly as possible.

Hippocrates (460–377 BCE)

As an intern at the county hospital, I was assigned to cover the plastic and burn surgery service every other night with about thirty floor patients and eight patients in the burn ICU. One evening, a young girl with significant burns in the ICU yanked out her tracheostomy (breathing tube). She was about to die, so I did not have time to put on the usual sterile gloves and gown to go into her room. I ran to her bed and put in her tube barehanded. Earlier that day, I had scrubbed on about five different skin graft cases and had unwittingly denuded a small area on one finger. My hand looked fine for a few days, but I developed a painful lump in my elbow. Several days later, I noticed a red streak running up my arm originating at my now obviously infected finger. I had inoculated my digit with bacteria when I inserted the young woman's tracheostomy tube without gloves. I had to be hospitalized for a week and was put on heavy-duty antibiotics to cure my resistant staph infection.

When I was in medical school, one of the surgical infectious disease faculty members used to take out the entire team to get margaritas and chips on Friday evenings. He was very senior and informed us that a particular type of infection, *pseudomonas*, "smelled like a wet corn tortilla." Decades later, while running the surgical ICU at another institution, I diagnosed this infection in a patient while on rounds using only my large proboscis and sense of smell. This amazed my critical care team. The medical students, who always kept us on our toes, challenged me by claiming that this organism, according to the textbook, should smell more like fruit jelly. "Nope," I responded. "A wet corn tortilla." But being an open-minded surgeon-scientist, I said we should investigate this question. We designed an experiment where we blindfolded three med students and had them smell actual *pseudomonas* along with multiple other substances, from fruit jelly to beer to wet corn tortillas. We used a scale of 0 to 10, with 10 smelling exactly like *pseudomonas*. What did we find? It turns out that the substance that smells precisely like *pseudomonas* is . . . *pseudomonas* itself (9.9 on the scale), with wet corn tortilla (9.4) close behind. No other substance was even a 5.0!

Other types of infections have odors, and the most unpleasant are the so-called mixed infections with multiple bacterial types. Think foul diarrhea. This can be overpowering during extensive operations with lots of pus. One learns to become a mouth breather in surgery to tolerate the stench when encountering big stinky situations (masks do not help).

The schnoz: While not immense, I do not think anyone would claim that I have a "button" nose. It is large and in charge. And, apparently, a near-lethal weapon, as you will learn. Some years ago, I was asked to talk at a national surgical conference on the subject of resistant staphylococcal infections (you may know them as MRSA). This type of infection is common in athletes from locker rooms (my daughter, Elizabeth, contracted it during high school basketball). The resistant type is already present in about two-thirds of folks we admit to the hospital with staph infections (a common cause of skin infections). Many people carry it asymptomatically in their noses, particularly hospital workers. A few months before my surgical conference, and allegedly during an errant kiss (my nose touched her orbit), I inoculated my wife, the Divine Ms. M. She first developed a sty under her eye, which spread to around her eye socket and then swarmed down her face in a matter of hours. She was transformed from a beauty to a beast (think Audrey Hepburn morphing into Quasimodo). I informed her that we needed to immediately head to the emergency room for intravenous antibiotics, as she had a case of facial cellulitis. After hours of waiting for confirmation of my diagnosis and a round of antibiotics, the condition receded. Ms. M. was disappointed that she could not attend the Tower of Power concert we had tickets to see that evening. Only later did I inform her how close she had come to being deathly ill. This condition can kill you if it spreads to your brain. Now she blames the "schnoz" for everything (even though there is no proof she got sick from my proboscis). I should mention that I refrained from showing any of the photographs of my dear wife looking like the Hunchback of Notre Dame with her facial cellulitis at my national conference, despite the urging of Ms. M.

If you hear hoofbeats, think horses, not zebras!

ANONYMOUS

As a senior medical student working at a medical clinic, I examined a man who had a rash on his lower leg. He was passing through from Louisiana to visit family and stated this rash had been there for a while and was bothersome. I observed a round lesion that looked like a circle of slightly raised red skin on the front of his shin. It must have triggered some deep memory of a class lecture a few years prior on infectious diseases. For some reason, I decided to touch the center of the rash and then probe it with a sharp object. No sensation at all. After a bit more questioning, I became convinced of my diagnosis. I walked out into the doctor's consultation area and announced that I had a patient with leprosy in my exam room. (According to the CDC, there are only about 150 cases of leprosy diagnosed each year in the United States and 250,000 worldwide. While it is a scary-sounding disease, it is not very contagious and is readily treatable with antibiotics.) After determining that I was not joking, I was swept away by the torrent of medical residents and then faculty. Suddenly, I was an onlooker to the brilliant diagnosis that they had made.

Early in training, we are advised to avoid looking at every symptom and sign of disease as a portent to some incredibly rare lesion or disease process. (So, better to seek "horses.") Searching for the bizarre and unusual (the "zebras") can be harmful to a patient who has a routine problem. It can lead to costly evaluation and unnecessary delays in patient management. A good example of this in the trauma field is cardiac contusion. As a resident, I admitted and managed countless patients with this diagnosis after car crashes whose elevated heart rate (and with it, a slight change in their electrocardiogram [ECG]) required overnight ICU admission. (Later it was demonstrated that there were no clinical consequences of this condition.) As a junior faculty member, I was involved in a study with some cardiologists that confirmed that unless there was a dangerous arrhythmia or cardiac pump failure (extremely unusual after trauma), none of these people had an actual cardiac injury. I was asked to prepare a lecture on the subject and found that there were more papers written on the topic at the time (over one hundred) than there were patients confirmed with this diagnosis. Many of the investigators that wrote the initial papers on the importance of the injury, ten years later wrote papers on its lack of importance. I can count on one hand the number of patients I have seen with an actual blunt cardiac injury after forty years in the field. One notable exception was a construction worker who was struck in the chest by a wrecking ball while on the job site. One of his coronary arteries was torn off, damaging his heart, but he survived. Now that is a true blunt cardiac injury! But a tremendous amount of work and hospital resources have gone into chasing this diagnosis in patients with minor chest trauma.

But occasionally, one stumbles onto something quite zebra-like. When I was an intern rotating on the medical service, I was asked to evaluate a patient who had arrived at the emergency room after a seizure. He had been seen repeatedly in the ER of our county hospital over the previous month with seizures following episodes where he had been observed staggering "drunk" about the neighborhood. Many alcoholics manifest seizure disorders from alcohol withdrawal or prior head trauma, but there was something strange about this story. First, he insisted he was only a social drinker. Reviewing his records from this and the prior admissions, what stood out was his very low blood sugar on each admission (less than 50, with normal being over 100), and zero blood alcohol. When I looked at his records from previous visits, he had always awakened quickly from his seizures and had been discharged expeditiously to the care of his family. When a patient has a seizure, the emergency medical technicians (EMTs) routinely inject an ampule of glucose just in case the patient has severely low glucose levels, which can mimic the appearance of drunkenness and, in severe cases, an epileptic seizure. Now, there is a very, very rare condition called an insulinoma, whereby a pancreatic tumor makes excess insulin, which causes the patient to have very low blood sugar. From what I can find in the literature, the incidence of insulinoma is about one to four cases per million in the general population. I called the surgical service with my presumed diagnosis, and they sprinted to the ER to see this man. Fortunately, his very unusual but aggressive tumor was successfully removed. Years later, I operated on a similar patient whose insulinoma was the size of a Ping-Pong ball and was wrapped in blood vessels. It looked like a jewelry piece surrounded by infrared beams in a Mission Impossible *movie. As we tied off each blood vessel, the patient's blood glucose levels progressively rose to normal (as we were preventing the insulin from the tumor from entering the circulation). These are bizarre tumors.*

5

SAVING LIVES

A gunshot wound is often not completely understood at first,
for it is at first, in many cases, impossible
to know what parts are killed.
JOHN HUNTER (1728–1793)

A dying seven-year-old boy arrived at the trauma center with a gunshot wound to the neck. He had been found in a home with thirty-two loaded weapons, unsupervised, and had been shot by his five-year-old sister. The bullet had crossed from the base of the neck across to the right lung and transected one of the main arteries to the brain, the left common carotid artery. We repaired this vessel with a sternotomy (the midline incision of the chest) and neck exploration, and he barely survived. About 1 percent of unintentional (accidental) gunshot wounds end in death. This is compared to the 5 to 20 percent mortality rate we see when looking at gunshot wounds overall.

In 1996, a short time after the massacre of thirty-five people in Tasmania, Australia enacted gun laws that led to a dramatic and sustained decrease in both gun-related homicides and suicides. In contrast, the response of the US Congress to the Australian massacre was to pass the NRA-supported Dickey Amendment in 1997, which cut funding to the CDC for gun-related research and put in regulations mandating that an institution would lose federal funding if it performed investigations on this subject.[1]

Not surprisingly, there has been extraordinarily little research on guns or the effects of gun control measures in the last twenty-five years in the United States. This appears to be the equivalent of what would have happened if the tobacco industry had successfully lobbied Congress in the 1960s to outlaw research on lung cancer and its relationship to smoking. If that had happened, would we understand today that smoking increases the incidence of cancer, along with heart disease and stroke?

America is number one in gun violence, with twenty times more gun-related deaths than any other country in the developed world. There were over one hundred mass shootings in the United States from 1996 to 2016, with more than five hundred deaths (and zero mass shootings in Australia). I am often asked my opinion on what can be done about the gun violence issue that affects us all in America. I answer that I am frankly ignorant because of an absence of research data in the United States. We lack information on the effectiveness of gun control measures such as the impact of assault rifles, magazine size, bullet type, and gun safety measures. And we remain ignorant regarding the importance of mental illness, concealed carry laws, and restricting the sale of weapons and their impact on gun-related injury. We have so many guns in the United States now (in 2018, estimated to be around 393.3 million), it is hard to know what measures would lower the incidence of firearm injuries and deaths. But it is clear that living in an armed nation requires many more safety measures.

In the early 1960s, car crashes were often fatal. Today, the United States has reduced the motor vehicle fatality rate by more than 500 percent due to multiple measures, including seat belts, airbags, divided highways, and vehicle redesign. We did not outlaw the driving of cars but rather made them safer for drivers and passengers. Amazingly, some states have made it illegal for a physician to even talk to a patient about gun safety. Yes, you read that correctly. From 2011 to 2017, when it was finally struck down, a Florida law prevented physicians (specifically pediatricians) from even discussing guns in the home with patient family members. If they ignored this law, they risked losing their medical license.

One of the worst experiences I ever had in trauma was the case of a three-year-old boy brought to the hospital after firing a loaded weapon he had found on the back seat of the family car. The child was dying on arrival with blood and brain matter pouring out of his skull, but we coded him (pumped on his chest and resuscitated him) for about an hour while his parents huddled at the head of the bed. When it became apparent to everyone that we could do no more, I pronounced the child dead. The mother let out a blood-curdling wail and started screaming at her husband as she pounded on his chest with her fists. The physicians and nurses scattered. The reality was that this drama was too much even for us hardened trauma veterans. It was a visceral reaction that we could all empathize with. It could have been one of our innocent children, lost to stupidity. I remember saying I wish I'd had a video of this episode to show to people who glorify the uncontrolled availability of the mighty gun.

I moved to the Southwest when my son was turning thirteen. I was deathly afraid of my boy, the wild man, being injured by an accidental discharge of a firearm. Guns are ubiquitous in that part of the country. So I bought a 22-gauge rifle and took him target shooting to learn about gun safety. On one of these outings, he discharged his weapon at the target until it failed to fire. "I'm out," Sam stated. "Did you clear the chamber?" I asked. "I counted, and I am empty," he responded authoritatively. I made him clear the weapon and out popped a live round. He turned pale. That experience was worth the price of the rifle.

> *The surgeon never suffers greater anxiety than*
> *when he is called upon to suppress a violent hemorrhage,*
> *and on no occasion is the reputation of his art*
> *so much at stake.*
>
> **JFD Jones (~1811)**

Late one night, a dying patient arrived at the trauma center by ambulance holding a bloody towel to her neck. Allegedly, she had been assaulted by her husband with a box cutter and feigned death for about twenty minutes, after which he left, and she was somehow able to call 911. We tried to reassure this terrified, wide-awake woman that all would be right. She was actively bleeding from her neck and was sucking air from the hole in her trachea. We placed an endotracheal (breathing) tube, held pressure on her neck, and transported her directly to the operating room. When I saw her in the office after the surgery—and also years later, when I testified at her attempted murder trial—I received a sincere "thank you" with a huge hug and some tears from the patient. She remembered every aspect of this horrible event, including her care in the trauma center. Even though we see them multiple times during their hospitalization (along with numerous other healthcare providers), our most serious trauma patients rarely have any idea who cared for them. Unfortunately, they are often unconscious and in dire straits on arrival. It makes us feel good in the rare instances when a patient appreciates our team's excellent care. Whenever I am thanked for saving someone's life, I always credit the entire team. Most of the time, they would have survived their trauma even without optimal care. But now and then, we do save a life.

Most of the trauma cases seen at some 450 trauma centers in the United States are blunt injuries sustained in falls, vehicle crashes, or workplace mishaps. How do we evaluate a fresh blunt trauma on arrival? Imagine that a person is stuffed into a large burlap bag and beaten severely by multiple people with baseball bats. The injured person is then removed from the bag, placed on a stretcher, and rolled into the emergency room. What are the injuries? The answer is, we have no idea. We take a standard approach as trauma surgeons to evaluate the injured, whether in a war zone or a civilian hospital. This approach is called the ABCs: Airway, Breathing, and Circulation. The woman mentioned above was at risk of bleeding to death from her neck wound and was also losing her airway and suffocating. In that case, we prioritized the airway in the trauma resuscitation area of the emergency room before heading up to the operating room to explore her neck wound while maintaining pressure on the wound to slow bleeding.

> *Gravity and dumbass keep us in business.*
> Anonymous

An older man arrived at the hospital in shock after falling from his ladder. He was trimming tree branches near his roof. After the initial resuscitation, the patient deteriorated and had a cardiac arrest. While the team was pumping on his chest, I went into the family area of the trauma center where this man's extended family had gathered. I told them that things looked very bleak. They responded that he had been brought in—having fallen while trimming this same tree and broken his back—one year prior. Gardening and tree trimming were his passions. We all agreed that at least he was doing something he loved in what turned out to be his last act.

So often, it is clear that injuries could have been avoided if some-one used their noggin. Like the guy cutting a tree branch 20 feet up while sitting on the branch (not kidding). Or putting a bullet in a vice and hitting it with a hammer. The list of "dumbass" things that folks do is endless. The tidal wave of trauma cases can be frustrating to the trauma care team. We in the field are dedicated to collaborating with the community to promote suc-cessful injury prevention programs such as those that address wearing seat belts and helmets. But we have failed in reducing other common causes of injury such as drunk driving and gun violence.

Much of what trauma centers across the United States treat are older adults falling from standing, from their bed, or down the stairs. They usually arrive with head injuries or rib or hip fractures and often show up with their bag of pills (and no one has any idea what they have ingested). Most older patients who end up on the ground inevitably have some form of bruise or laceration. The pre-hospital providers (EMTs and paramedics) cannot distinguish between a trauma patient and someone who has "gone to ground" after they sustained a heart attack, stroke, or any illness leading to a loss of consciousness. Said another way, just because you felt bad and laid down on the ground, you did not necessarily fall and sustain an injury. So all these folks arrive as potential traumas. We recently reviewed our trauma center experience and found that only about two in thirty geriatric patients who arrive after falls were admitted for injuries. Thus, nearly all older patients who experience falls go home with no trauma found.

The other interface we have with older patients at the trauma center is when folks continue to drive despite the fragility associated with medical illness, as this next story demonstrates. We were rounding in the ICU on a woman in her eighties who had been severely injured after the car she was riding in crashed at highway speeds. She was, fortunately, doing better than her husband, who had been at the wheel. He remained in the ICU and was being treated for irregular heartbeats and multiple episodes of ventricular tachycardia, an arrhythmia that can be associated with sudden death. When we told her about her partner's cardiac issues, she stated that this explained the actions of the previous few months. It seems that while driving, he would suddenly slump over, and she would need to "wake him up" by punching him in the chest. She had unknowingly been giving him what we call a precordial thump and jolting (essentially shocking) him out of this malignant rhythm.

According to US Census projections, the number of Americans sixty-five and older is expected to nearly double from fifty-two million in 2018 to ninety-five million by 2060. The sixty-five-and-older age group's share of the total population will rise from 16 percent to 23 percent. We often see old folks falling and banging their head and body, resulting in brain injuries and rib and hip fractures. When they drive a car, really bad things can happen. There is even a condition called SAE, which stands for "sudden acceleration of the elderly." This is a real thing: an older person jams their foot on the gas pedal rather than the brake and motors through an intersection or into a parked vehicle. This can be dangerous if someone is in the path of the careening vehicle. I have taken care of many older patients who have been run over by their own cars. This occurs when one exits the driver's seat with the engine running and the car still in gear. These injuries can be quite severe, particularly in frail older patients with multiple preexisting medical issues. Unfortunately, taking away a person's driver's license or even their vehicle because they are deemed unsafe to drive is problematic and associated with a lot of resistance. The automobile represents independence to folks in most regions of the United States (outside of New York City).

A good example of this dilemma was experienced by yours truly when my beloved grandmother Rosie was eighty-eight years old. Having just cared for several older people involved in driving disasters as the chief of trauma at a busy trauma center, I returned to Northern California to visit her at her apartment. Typically, I drove her to a nice lunch in her car. She owned a 1965 Pontiac Bonneville (one of the longest cars ever made). It was painted a metallic light green and was covered with large gray spots where a body shop had banged out large dents and then applied primer following contact with many different stationary objects. The car resembled a huge leopard poised for mayhem. Because Rosie had abrasions on her legs from falling on the single stair at the entrance of her apartment building, I was concerned that she was too wobbly to be driving. She was also blind as a bat. Later that evening, I discussed this issue with my parents at their house. They responded in unison: "You tell her." So I took a deep breath and called her to suggest that we needed to retire her car, as it was unsafe for her to drive. She was naturally really upset, despite my offer to get her taxi vouchers so she could manage her affairs. She only drove to the doctor's office (which was my father) and my parents' house anyway. The next day, she called me all excited. Her nephew Hal (he was in his seventies) was going to get her a used Cadillac. "No, Rosie, you don't understand, you should not be driving yourself anymore," I said. Silence. Then she said, "You just don't want me to drive!" "Correct," I responded. She never forgot that I (her favorite, and only, grandchild) had taken away her car for the remaining seven years of her life. But I think she forgave me.

> *I used to think that drinking was bad for me.*
> *So, I gave up thinking.*
>
> **ANONYMOUS**

On vacation during my senior year of medical school, I was driving up to ski in Lake Tahoe when the car's sea-level-adjusted carburetor stalled the engine on a two-lane road. I pulled over and off to the shoulder. I reached under the hood to open the butterfly valve of my mother's Oldsmobile Omega. My girlfriend started up the car; I closed the hood and hopped into the driver's seat. A split second later, we were struck by a Ford Econoline van at high speed. Our midsize car exploded. The windows burst; the front bench seat snapped off as we hurtled over 100 feet into a ditch. I extracted myself and my girlfriend from the car and then checked on the van driver, whom I could see was dazed. But as I approached, he exited the scene in his vehicle. The highway patrol recognized the van driver by my description and went to pick him up. He was driving drunk

*with a revoked license. If he had struck our vehicle a few seconds earlier,
I would have been killed instantly.*

One of the primary obstacles to injury prevention is driving while
under the influence, which, according to the CDC, accounts for
about 30 percent of vehicle-related deaths. So, about ten thousand
of the approximately thirty-five thousand vehicle-related deaths each
year in the United States are related to drunk driving. Every day,
thirty-two people in the United States die in motor vehicle crashes
that involve an alcohol-impaired driver. This has changed little in
the last thirty-five years despite various public campaigns. According
to the National Highway Traffic Safety Administration (NHTSA),
"Alcohol-involved crashes resulted in 14,219 fatalities, 497,000
injuries, and $68.9 billion in economic costs in 2019, accounting
for 20 percent of all crash costs."[2] (These losses include medical
costs, lost productivity, legal and court costs, emergency service
costs, insurance administration costs, congestion costs, property
damage, and workplace losses.) In 2016, more than one million
drivers were arrested for driving under the influence of alcohol or
narcotics. That is about 1 percent of the 111 million self-reported
episodes of alcohol-impaired driving among US adults each year.

What can we, as trauma surgeons, do about this? In addition
to advocating for stricter enforcement of existing laws, there is a
simple intervention in the hospital with an injured, intoxicated
person that can have a significant impact of long duration. A short
interaction with a trained professional (about fifteen or twenty
minutes of counseling, typically with a trauma social worker or
another expert in this area) has been shown by researchers to
reduce the likelihood of another alcohol-related injury and even

improve the patient's overall quality of life after the hospitalization, specifically, weekly alcohol use and binge-drinking episodes.[3] These improved outcomes were maintained over a forty-eight-month follow-up period. Investigators also found that those receiving this brief intervention experienced 20 percent fewer ER visits, 22 percent fewer nonfatal injuries, 37 percent fewer hospitalizations, 46 percent fewer arrests, and 50 percent fewer motor vehicle crashes. Essentially, the Screening, Brief Intervention, and Referral to Treatment (SBIRT) protocol helps an injured patient understand and practice avoidance of alcohol-related dangerous behaviors that can stem from drinking and driving.

These interventions, however, are not effective among the subset of drivers who have chronic alcohol dependence, about 6 percent of all drinkers. These "professional" drinkers often arrive at the ER after operating a vehicle with blood alcohol concentrations in the stratosphere, five to seven times the legal limit, which could kill an average person or put them in a coma. On more than one occasion, I asked one of these pickled people how much they drank, only to be told they had quit. When I asked one man, "When did you quit?" he said, "On the way to the hospital in the ambulance."

Any fool can cut off an arm or leg but
it takes a surgeon to save one.

GEORGE C. ROSS (1834–1892)

A fortyish Russian ice-skating coach was standing on a street corner when she was struck by an out-of-control car. She arrived at the ER in shock with a degloving injury of her entire leg (think peeled-off skin). Her leg bones were shattered in multiple places, and she had no pulses in her foot. The trauma team went into action, ruling out other injuries, and then she was brought to the operating room for care by multiple collaborating surgical services. There was serious consideration of whether this mangled leg needed to be amputated. The soft tissues and bones were severely damaged, including her blood vessels, but her nervous sensation was intact. The decision was to try to save the leg, and she underwent repair of her torn blood vessels and stabilization of the bones. But how were we to deal with the loss of skin? A new wound product was employed, which involves using the patient's skin cells to grow new skin and cover the leg. This woman was one of several success stories of patients who benefited from a skin autograft. A small piece of the patient's skin was removed and sent to a lab, where skin cells were extracted. Forty-eight hours later, the new skin-derived product was placed in a paste that was smeared on her wound (like cream cheese on a bagel). From this concoction grew tissue that resembled the native skin. After a few weeks under a dressing, voilà, new skin. Amazingly, within a year, she was back skating on the ice.

Most people mistakenly think that being shot by an assault rifle or crashing a car are the worst trauma mechanisms, but they are not. The worst mechanism of injury in the civilian world is being struck by a vehicle as a pedestrian. Military wounds with high-velocity weapons currently have a mortality rate of around 10 percent, and car crashes are significantly lower. Fifteen percent of pedestrians struck by a car will die, and the death rate is over 30 percent for older people. We see some horrific injuries when people are struck by vehicles. It is a matter of a 150-pound human versus 2,500 pounds of hurtling metal. The injuries typically involve multiple organ groups. Recently, we cared for an older man who was injured when a car went off the road above and landed on him as he worked in his backyard garden. His pelvic bone sheared through his urethra and rectum, and he came close to dying.

Years ago, my colleagues and I identified a major problem with a high frequency of children being struck by cars in South Florida. In investigations worldwide, children have similar constellations of injuries when struck by vehicles. Toddlers typically crawl under a wheel or stand up and get whacked in the head by a fender. Grade-school kids who live in densely populated, high-traffic neighborhoods classically run out into the street after a ball and are hit. Our immortal teenagers are hurt when car surfing (riding on the top of moving vehicles) or running corner to corner in busy intersections. In our investigations, we plotted the location of some five hundred kids struck by cars over three years and found that about half were injured near their elementary schools. Our group then constructed an intervention project working with various community organizations to lower the rates of children struck. We showed we could dramatically reduce the number of kids injured (think tenfold) and ultimately expanded the program to involve schoolchildren in the entire state.

One of the problems with injury prevention programs is they often require financial support from grants, so when the grant is completed and the money's gone, the program is over. Other programs depend on local taxes. When the program succeeds and eliminates the targeted injuries, the local or state government cuts the funding as if there is no longer a potential risk. We made sure our "Walk Safe" program worked and essentially cost nothing. This program includes a proven educational course for children, integrates law enforcement measures and school reengineering, and collaborates with parents and teachers. Two decades later, this project continues to prevent injuries among children in the state of Florida.

An injury to the head is never so slight as to be despised and never so severe as to be despaired of.

HIPPOCRATES (460–377 BCE)

A young man arrived at the ER by helicopter after crashing his motorcycle at highway speeds. He was wearing leathers and a full-face helmet. The paramedics had removed his helmet, which accompanied him to the trauma center. The side of the helmet was buffed down by contact with the roadway through the metal. He would have left part of his skull and brain on the street had he not been wearing a helmet. The patient sustained only a concussion.

The best way to lower morbidity (complications) and mortality (deaths) from injuries is to avoid trauma in the first place. Each trauma center has a program directed at avoiding trauma in its community. In the late 1950s, the value of the seat belt was established, and laws were imposed at the state level. The deaths per mile driven dramatically decreased over the next few decades from over six per 100 million miles driven to around one per 100 million miles driven today. Speed limits, divided roadways, and vehicle alterations (such as collapsible steering columns) have been significant factors in lowering mortality rates. Advanced techniques in the prehospital systems with more expertise among the ambulance crews and standardized medical care at receiving hospitals with rapid transfer to regional trauma centers have also had a profound impact.

According to the NHTSA, nearly half (47 percent) of the 22,215 passenger vehicle occupants killed in 2019 were not wearing seat belts (meaning, half of those who experienced trauma deaths might have survived if they had been wearing a seat belt). Seat belts saved an estimated 14,955 lives in 2017 alone. Wearing a seat belt keeps you in the vehicle and is required (and worn by more than 90 percent of drivers) in all states except New Hampshire (in line with the state's motto, "Live free or die"). The likelihood of a significant injury or death if you are ejected from a moving vehicle is many times higher. For example, if you take flight out of your car, the chance of a significant injury to your cervical vertebrae (skeletal bones of your neck) is almost 10 percent. In addition to securing you inside the vehicle, seat belts work by slowing your deceleration rate. If you strike the dashboard, you are moving at a reduced speed. This minimizes the amount of kinetic energy absorbed by your noggin.

There is, however, a constellation of injuries related to wearing seat belts, typically in high-impact collisions. Of course, you would probably be dead without the restraint as you smashed into the dashboard or flew out the window. When a person is secured by the seat belt, specific organs, such as the small intestine, bladder, and pancreas, can be compressed between the belt and the spine. Points of fixation in the chest, such as the aorta shortly after it exits the heart, and in the abdomen, such as where the bowel is attached, can tear. Following a really bad car crash, these seat belt–related injuries in a surviving patient are much preferable to an inevitable death.

*Failure to promptly recognize and treat simple life-threatening
injuries is the tragedy of trauma, not the inability to handle
the catastrophic or complicated injury.*

F. WILLIAM BLAISDELL (1927–2020)

*The call was to the urology service, which I was covering as an intern for
the county hospital, regarding a motorcycle rider who had crashed and
could not urinate. The patient had been transferred to us from an outlying hospital after a negative "wallet biopsy" (not having sufficient funds
or insurance). They had placed a urinary catheter without obtaining any
urine and sent him to us. In the days before the Emergency Medical Treatment and Labor Act (EMTALA) law against dumping (sending patients
without providing care because of their limited financial resources), individuals were frequently transferred without the acceptance of the receiving hospital. (EMTALA is a federal law that requires anyone coming to
an emergency department to be stabilized and treated, regardless of their
ability to pay, since its enactment in 1986.) When I found the patient in
the corner of the emergency room, he was agitated with an extreme need
to pee. I looked at the empty urinary bag. The catheter had been shoved
into his penis, but it exited from a cut in his perineum (base of his penis),
where he had likely struck the gas cap as he straddled the crashing motorcycle. So the catheter never entered his bladder but was lying between his
legs with the balloon inflated. Now, after an infusion of liters of fluid at
the sending hospital and en route to us, the patient was ready to burst. I
placed a suprapubic tube straight into his bladder for relief. The patient
now faced the prospect of major reconstructive surgery on his urethra.*

The risk of death for motorcyclists in accidents is thirty times
greater than for car drivers and passengers. As a former motorcycle

rider, it became clear to me that you must continuously ride as if you are invisible to other motorists (and I always rode in full gear). Three-quarters of all motorcycle deaths occur at low speeds (30 miles per hour or less) in residential areas. That is because the enemy of the motorcycle rider is not so much the ground as it is the car. For automobiles, approximately 31 percent of crashes result in injury, but only 0.3 percent of collisions are fatal. Eighty percent of reported crashes result in injury for motorcycles, and about 4.4 percent of crashes are fatal. Even when helmets are worn, the devastating injuries to the rest of the body that can occur when it is struck by a car can be complex to manage. Recently, I cared for a young man whose pelvis had been crushed in a low-speed motorcycle crash. He bled severely and required a massive transfusion. The orthopedic service quickly stabilized his pelvic bones after our team of angiographers (the radiologists that use special catheters to block bleeding arteries) occluded some bleeding pelvic vessels. I explored the abdomen to address some additional bleeding. Fortunately, everything went smoothly, and after some 30 units of blood and multiple orthopedic operations, he survived to go to rehab. With plans to sell his motorcycle . . .

Helmets prevent serious brain injury and save lives whether the vehicle is a bicycle or a motorcycle. A study performed in Seattle in the 1990s found that bicycle helmets reduced the risk of severe brain injury by 85 percent.[4] In most states, bicycle helmets are required only for children. Unfortunately, in the mid-1970s, the federal government withdrew highway funds that had supported the law requiring people to wear a motorcycle helmet. Many states repealed their motorcycle helmet laws in response, and there was a substantial increase in severe head trauma cases after motorcycle crashes. You usually do not die when you crash your motorcycle without a helmet, nor do you become an organ donor. Rather, after a long, expensive hospital course, you end up unresponsive, in a permanent vegetative state for the rest of your days—breathing out of your neck while receiving tube feeding. Most people do not realize that the taxpayer bears the costs of these devastating brain injuries, as essentially no one's insurance pays for this level of long-term disability. And we are talking many billions of dollars per year.

The freedom to "feel the asphalt through your hair" must be balanced with the prohibitive cost to society. I was in Florida in July 2000 when state legislators slipped a law by the trauma community that eliminated the state motorcycle helmet requirement. These local representatives responded to their constituents who demanded the liberty to ride helmetless. The state's antihelmet crusade leader ironically died later that month after a motorcycle crash. She was not wearing a helmet . . .

> *To refuse to treat any aneurysm . . . is unwise, but it is also*
> *dangerous to operate upon all of them.*
>
> ANTYLLUS (SECOND CENTURY CE)

After a high-speed crash, a morbidly obese young man high on cocaine and alcohol arrived at a community hospital. After about six hours of evaluation there, we were called to accept the transfer, as he could not fit on their CT scanner. On arrival at our facility, our examination and imaging revealed blood in his chest consistent with an aortic transection, essentially a traumatic aneurysm (a partial tear of this large blood vessel). An angiogram confirmed this, and he was rushed to the operating room,

where one of our cardiothoracic surgeons attempted to repair his aorta.
Unfortunately, it was too late, and he could not be revived. Despite
everything being done quickly and correctly at our institution, the sur-
geon and hospital were sued. I was later named in the lawsuit (which
was dropped) because the cardiac surgeon had passed away from a medi-
cal illness.

Trauma centers get extremely busy with vehicular crashes, particularly motorcycle crashes, when the weather improves, especially
in summer. Even gunshot wounds seem to escalate in the swelter-
ing summer months. This is not the case in South Florida, which
experiences mostly the same volume of trauma cases every month,
because the temperature is fairly consistent all year long. But the
increase is typical of the Northeast, where folks hibernate in the
winter months. The problem for trauma surgeons is that the kids
are out of school during the summer, and we want to enjoy family
vacations like everyone else. But that is when it is superbusy, and
we need lots of surgical backup. For example, on one Fourth of
July in the Northeast some years ago, I saw four severely injured
patients with blunt thoracic aortic tears (an unusual injury to the
main blood vessel that exits the heart, commonly associated with
extremely high-energy trauma). At that institution, we typically saw
that many aortic injuries total from Labor Day to Memorial Day.

There seems to be a significant decrease in trauma (particularly that of penetrating violence) during certain times of the year.
We expect to see a reduction in activity during important holidays
(like Christmas and Thanksgiving) when everyone hangs out with
their family members. When folks are watching the Super Bowl,
the World Series, the NBA finals, and the World Cup soccer final,

the trauma center is often dead-quiet. We were unsuccessful in validating this in a research study because it was hard to figure out when to start the clock before and after the sporting events. While it is certainly not a proven thing, it does seem like trauma slows down when people are busy watching sports or having major holiday gatherings. I can report that during the final episode of *Game of Thrones*, we noticed that there appeared to be hardly a car moving on the streets of Manhattan.

6

DEALING WITH THE WORST INJURIES

*Injection of fluid that will increase blood pressure
has dangers in itself. Hemorrhage in a case of shock may not have
occurred to a marked degree because blood pressure has been too
low and the flow too scant to overcome the obstacle offered
by the clot. If the pressure is raised before the surgeon is ready to
check any bleeding that may take place, blood that is sorely
needed may be lost.*

WALTER B. CANNON (1871–1945)

*It was a sunny snow day, and the man had spent the morning sledding
with his family. On one run, he crashed into a tree. This big, burly guy
decided to tough it out and watch football despite some pain. In the evening, he felt faint when he stood up, and his wife insisted on bringing
him to the emergency room. On arrival, he was talking but had a low
blood pressure. In those days (more than thirty years ago), the standard
management of hypotension was to infuse massive amounts of fluids and
drive up the blood pressure to normal. As the surgeon on call for the
trauma center that night, I was informed that this young man was
receiving fluids and had a bloody tap (blood was aspirated from the*

abdominal space). We planned to rush him to the operating room to perform an emergency abdominal exploration. I arrived from home in fifteen minutes and found the patient dead on a stretcher next to the OR table. His heart had stopped in the elevator.

For about fifty years, starting in the early 1960s, it was standard practice to give bleeding trauma patients massive amounts of fluids. We would typically place a few large intravenous catheters and have various support staff squeeze in the contents of liter bags of fluid. This fluid was saline or lactated Ringer's solution, which is full of electrolytes but lacks the ability to carry oxygen as blood does. This infusion would raise the patient's blood pressure, which was thought to be beneficial to avoid poor organ perfusion. Of course, the body's normal physiological response to bleeding is to lower blood pressure and create clots to stop the hemorrhage (tamponade). Subsequent studies, first in animal models and then in patients, demonstrated that raising the blood pressure with ongoing and uncontrolled bleeding was harmful. Today, because of the advances in our knowledge, the patient mentioned above might have survived. The current approach is to gently infuse blood and blood products and delay raising the blood pressure until we control the bleeding (in this case, removing the patient's ruptured spleen during abdominal exploratory surgery). During World War I, this concept was proposed (see quote above from Cannon, which he wrote in 1918), but it took us a century to recognize the wisdom and adopt this as standard practice in the resuscitation of our trauma patients. Why? Because there is still significant resistance in medicine to challenging the dogma of the day. One physician survey revealed that the type of fluid physicians administer to critically ill patients was related to when they were trained and what they were instructed to infuse during their residency. Adoption of change is slow.

All bleeding eventually ceases.

GUY DE CHAULIAC (1300–1368)

The medical condition known as shock was best described in the 1800s by physicians Samuel Gross and John C. Warren as the "rude unhinging of the machinery of life." Your organs do not get enough oxygen and start to fail. If you do not restore oxygen delivery to meet the demands of the cells, the organs and the patient die. Most clinicians would agree that if a patient has a significant trauma mechanism, clinically looks like they are bleeding, requires blood transfusions, and then develops organ failure, they are in shock.

It is not always clear who qualifies as a patient suffering from shock. Years ago, I received a call from an outlying hospital about a young man with a gunshot wound to the groin. He was actively bleeding and had a systolic blood pressure of 60 millimeters of mercury (mmHg); normal is around 120mmHg. I told the sending physician that this patient might not survive the transport. He responded, "Probably." We sent a helicopter crew on a three-hour round trip to the hospital. They transfused 4 units of blood on the return leg of the journey. The patient arrived cold, with no blood pressure, but he had a barely palpable carotid pulse. He had nearly completely bled out. We rushed him to the operating room for a massive transfusion and abdominal exploration. There is a scene in the movie Black Hawk Down *in which an army ranger dies from bleeding after a bullet strikes his groin. That was the type of injury that we controlled in the operating room. The hardest part of managing this type of vascular injury is getting control of the bleeding. In this case, after clamping off the abdominal aorta, we repaired the lacerated right common iliac artery (the major blood vessel to the leg). We returned to the OR the next day to close his abdominal wound. The patient had no complications and went home five days later. By the strict definition above, as he had no organ dysfunction, he had not been in shock. But it does sound like we need to get some of his DNA and replicate him. And he should stay away from kryptonite.*

Blood is a very special juice.

JOHANN WOLFGANG VON GOETHE (1749–1832)

Crossing the circular driveway entrance to the university hospital to see his cardiologist, an older gentleman was struck by a taxicab. He was essentially hurled through the emergency room doors. The ER team wrapped his head in a huge gauze dressing to cover his large scalp laceration and let him sit in the waiting area for a few hours. (This, unfortunately, occurs often in our overcrowded emergency rooms.) Then the surgical team was consulted to care for this man who had bled in the ER and was now in a state of shock. He had saturated the turban of gauze with units of blood and had a profound drop in blood pressure.

About half of the folks who arrive at the hospital after trauma, having hemorrhaged to the degree that they have a low blood pressure, do so from what we call noncavitary bleeding. This is blood loss that is not "internal" bleeding into the thoracic or abdominal cavities but instead comes from a laceration (the scalp is a frequent site) or broken bones. Anyone who has done a first aid course knows that the first response is always to apply pressure and terminate bleeding. Some injuries are less amenable to stopping with pressure, however. The scalp will often bleed significantly unless it is sutured or staples are applied. When a patient arrives with a bloody dressing or a head covered in blood, we quickly assess them from head to toe and then close the wounds. Even taking a patient for a quick head CT can give them time to bleed pints of blood from an untreated scalp laceration. We probably see more actively bleeding scalp lacerations than any other wound, as most of the others will stop when EMTs apply a compression dressing.

As a chief resident, I was helping a junior resident repair a hernia when a nurse charged into the room and shouted that they needed me immediately (stat) in another operating room. I told my assistant to hit the pause button and that I would return soon. As I stepped into the hallway, I could see a trail of blood leading from the elevator down the corridor, and I followed it into an operating room. The resident team was about to prep this patient with a stab wound to the neck for surgery. A medical student held a huge wad of blood-saturated towels and gauze pads on the patient's neck, and there was blood leaking everywhere. I told him to step back, remove all the bloody mess of dressing materials, and place a single finger on the bleeding site. Once the bleeding had ceased, we could prepare the site, get adequate exposure, and explore the neck. A few sutures in the blood vessel were all that was required.

> *The transition between life and death*
> *should be gentle in the winter of life.*
>
> RUDOLPH MATAS (1860–1957)

A ninety-two-year-old woman fell and struck her neck on the edge of the bathtub, crushing her upper cervical vertebrae and transecting her spinal cord. Her son was present and immediately started mouth-to-mouth resuscitation, and someone called 911. High spinal cord injuries damage the nerve supply to the diaphragm and therefore prevent one's ability to breathe, so most folks sustaining this trauma die at the scene of the injury. In this case, the patient survived and was mentally intact. The life span of an older patient with a high spinal cord injury is very short, and mechanical ventilation is required. During a family meeting, this patient clearly indicated that she did not want to go on with life as a permanently paralyzed, ventilator-dependent quadriplegic. Present with many of the patient's relatives was a compassionate team of doctors, nurses, and social workers. The family left the ICU room and promptly told the stunned critical care team that they were "murderers" (although no measures to end the patient's life had been taken) and transferred the patient to another hospital.

Older people tend to fare worse than younger trauma victims with the same constellation of injuries. This is primarily because older individuals recover poorly from brain injuries. A young person can survive a severe brain injury that would devastate an older person. For example, Joseph, one of my surgical interns (in his twenties), was on a bike ride with his friends and fell, bumping his head. The following day, he did not show up for work. One of his fellow interns went by Joseph's residence and found him unconscious. He was rushed to the hospital and then to the operating room for emergency brain surgery. He underwent drainage of his large epidural hematoma (a significant brain bleed that typically results from a severed artery after a skull fracture). Joseph recovered, finished his residency program, and became a leading plastic surgeon in the Northeast. If an eighty-year-old had this same injury, they would likely not awaken following surgery. The family would be faced with the choice of long-term care with a minimal chance of meaningful recovery or withdrawal of life support.

The other complicating issue in older people is preexisting medical conditions and medications. Unlike some countries where medication history is readily available to all healthcare providers in a national database, patients often arrive at trauma centers in the United States with no medication history or with just a big bag of pill bottles. We often have no idea what the patient is actually ingesting. The drugs that make our lives most difficult in trauma care are blood thinners. These cause the patient's blood clotting to be abnormal and can lead to more bleeding. An enormous number of older Americans are taking blood thinners. The newer blood thinners like Eliquis, Pradaxa, and Xarelto can be difficult to reverse. Meaning the antidote to these blood thinners, which would help make the patient clot normally after an injury, is expensive and not widely available. (For example, the only approved reversal agent is Andexxa, which costs $58,000 per reversal dose.) But not knowing if patients are on anticoagulation medication when they arrive means that they continue to bleed while we perform various tests to detect a clotting abnormality that we can reverse. Remember, these folks often appear without family or any information, so we do not know what injury they have sustained (like a brain bleed) and have no idea if they are taking blood thinners that require a reversal agent.

> *Life is short, and art long; the crisis fleeting,*
> *experience perilous, and decision difficult.*
>
> HIPPOCRATES (460–377 BCE)

I was talking to a seemingly intoxicated man who had been transported from the scene of a bad car crash. As he rolled into the trauma room, he was very belligerent. I asked if he had any recollection of the event. "Yes," he said, "I remember everything perfectly. That SOB . . . cut me off in the intersection and . . ." He then stopped speaking and blew a pupil (a widely dilated and unequal—blown—pupil is a sign of pressure on the brain and a potential catastrophe). He was rushed to head CT and then to the OR for emergent decompression of his bleeding brain.

Each year, two to three million folks in the United States have minor head injuries resulting in a temporary loss of consciousness (or a concussion). Many of these injuries are sports related. More importantly, 225,000 Americans sustain a significant head injury, and about sixty thousand die from brain trauma each year. The leading causes of these traumatic brain injuries are falls and motor vehicle crashes. The population of older people is at particular risk for sustaining significant head injury. They are prone to falling and often have conditions that require medications that prevent clotting. A pet peeve of mine is when someone states that the patient "denies loss of consciousness." As the above exemplifies, folks who are knocked out (rendered unconscious) do not remember it. They may have a brief period of consciousness during which they (and sometimes the health provider) are confused as to what occurred.

We use the Glasgow Coma Score (GCS) to assess motor, verbal, and eye-opening responses to stimuli. This allows providers to communicate about mental acuity using a commonly employed assessment tool. A normal GCS is 15. Anything below 9 is considered a profound decrease in cognitive function (a coma, in lay terms) and usually warrants support by a ventilator. The lowest possible GCS is 3. Patients who are physiologically stable and have a persistent GCS of 3 are evaluated for brain death. If there is no evidence of any brain stem activity (the most basic of the brain functions), such as spontaneous breathing or gag reflex, and if the patient meets strict physiological criteria, they undergo an apnea test. The patient is disconnected from the ventilator for about fifteen minutes, during which time they are monitored for respiratory activity. They are declared brain dead if they do not breathe during the apnea exam. We are required by law to notify the organ donor network, and the family is contacted for potential organ donation, if appropriate.

As providers, dealing with families after their loved ones have undergone a declaration of brain death is often a nightmare. Next of kin often do not believe the clinician's diagnosis of brain death. They see that the patient is not responding but the heart is still beating. And once reality has set in, it is not unusual for the family to feel guilty because they allowed their sixteen-year-old to ride his Kawasaki 500 motorcycle intoxicated and without a helmet, or failed to keep a loaded gun out of the hands of their toddler, resulting in the child's brain death. And even when there is a clearly expressed desire by the patient (even in writing) to be an organ donor, it is not unusual for families to override the patient's wishes, thus depriving six or more potential recipients of a precious lifesaving new organ. In some countries like Spain, organ donation is an opt-out culture, meaning that legally, everyone is an organ donor unless otherwise specified. The rates of organ donation in these countries are about double those of opt-in countries such as the United States.[1]

Of course, not all brain injuries are as they initially appear. During my fellowship training, a patient was brought into the hospital with apparent major brain trauma. He was found by the paramedics lying unresponsive under a park bench late one night. They noted some questionable bruising of the head in the dim light. They attempted to intubate (insert a breathing tube) without success. The patient arrived at the ER still unresponsive, so when the trauma team could not intubate the patient either, they cut a hole in his neck (called an emergency cricothyroidotomy) to secure his airway. It is routine to establish an airway in patients with very depressed mental activity to ensure they will not stop breathing. The patient then underwent a CT scan of the head, which revealed evidence of prior head trauma of questionable age. With his continued low level of responsiveness (apparent deep coma), we felt that it was prudent to insert a monitor into his skull to measure brain pressure (standard in those days). In the morning, our patient awoke from his severe alcohol intoxication, and, pointing to the pressure monitor in his skull and the tube in his neck, he mouthed, "What the f---?" The lesson here is to avoid getting too drunk and passing out on the Boston Common.

> *The heart is the chief mansion of the soul, the organ of vital capacity, the beginning of life, the foundation of the vital spirits . . . the first to live and the last to die.*
>
> **AMBROISE PARÉ (1510–1590)**

A young man arrived at the trauma center with a woman's hairbrush stuck in his left chest, right over his heart. The handle was embedded to the hilt, with the cylindrical brush abutting the skin. The brush pulsated with each heartbeat because the end was inside the heart.

Stab wounds are certainly not as lethal as gunshot wounds (about one-third of the death rate), but they are all about location. One patient arrived at the ER facedown with a huge knife jammed between his scapula and ribs. He could not lift his arm or turn over, but the blade had missed all critical structures. Another patient arrived at the emergency room with a 7-inch knife rammed all the way to the handle between their eyes but miraculously sustained no brain injury. Both survived. Just like in real estate, it's location, location, location!

Patients with stab wounds usually present with just a hole in their skin, not attached to the actual knife. Thus, we have no idea about the size of the blade or what underlying organ may be injured. For example, a huge man, 6 feet, 5 inches and 250 pounds, arrived at the trauma center with a small hole in his left armpit and stable vital signs. During his routine evaluation, we found that he had a laceration of his heart, which was a good 15 inches away from the hole. Had he been stabbed with a sword?

Penetrating wounds (gunshots or knife wounds) to the thorax are particularly dangerous, as injuries to the heart can be very subtle. Only about 25 percent of cardiac wounds have any symptoms. Cardiac tamponade occurs when the normally empty space around the heart (called the pericardial sac) becomes filled with fluid and prevents blood from returning to the heart. With each heartbeat, more blood squirts out of the heart into this space through the wound and makes it even harder for the heart to work. Eventually, the heart stops, and the patient dies. We call the rectangular space between the top and bottom of the breastplate in the center of the torso the "zone of death." Anything entering or potentially traversing this space (in the case of the gunshot wound) could result in a cardiac wound and therefore requires meticulous investigation.

Two memorable chest injury stories involve survivors. In one case (courtesy of Steven Brower, M.D.), a young man arrived in the ER after a stab to the chest and promptly had a cardiac arrest. The senior resident "cracked his chest," performing an emergency thoracotomy right in the trauma room. He opened the chest from the edge of the breastplate to the spine and evacuated blood from the pericardium, and the heart started to beat again. This was done immediately on arrival with no time to place a breathing tube or give any medications. The patient was in profound shock, and there was no time for anesthesia. With the heart now pumping away, the patient woke up and sat up on the stretcher. As he viewed his open chest and pounding heart, he yelled, "Call my mama." He survived, and we did.

The second story involves a young man who arrived at the trauma center in shock with multiple bullet wounds to the chest. We were able to get him to the operating room, where we opened his left chest and repaired some holes in his heart. He still had a low blood pressure, so we opened his abdomen from the breastplate to the pelvis to find a liver injury that was not bleeding. The patient continued to be in profound shock from bleeding, but we could not locate the source. So we opened the middle of the chest in a sternotomy and then the right chest horizontally to find the bleeding point. It was in an extremely tough spot, just above the diaphragm in the back of the main blood vessel to the heart, the vena cava. Amazingly, this patient survived, a rare event with an injury in this location. About six months later, he returned to the clinic complaining that he was a Muslim and the surgeons had carved the sign of the crucifix on his body. He was unaware that his surgeon was Jewish and that he was probably the only person on the planet to have that scar and live to talk about it.

Those who do not feel pain seldom think that it is felt.

Samuel Johnson (1709–1784)

I crashed while skiing below the summit on a steep, icy mountain section. I had decided to buy a new set of ski boots on this trip but had rented a pair for the first day that were, in retrospect, too big. When my feet shrunk in the cold, I slid around in the boots and lost my grip. Usually, a fall is no big deal, but I somehow managed to land on my ski pole. I could not catch a full breath and knew this was trouble. My friends called for ski patrol, but I decided I could ski down. A chest X-ray at the base aid station revealed a flail chest, which is when the ribs are broken in a few places and the chest wall moves opposite to the direction it is supposed to. When you inhale, your chest is sucked in rather than expanding. Off I went to the trauma center. On arrival, they figured out I was a surgeon and asked me for directions on my care, which I declined to give. "Do your usual workup, but I can pee," I said to avoid a urinary catheter. They then inadvertently rolled me over onto the crushed side of my chest, which certainly got my attention. The primary treatment for chest wall injury is just pain control and deep breathing exercises. So the following day I returned to the ski lodge, where I spent the rest of the trip trying not to laugh or sneeze, both of which hurt like the devil. My favorite thing was the loud crunching sound emanating from my chest that could be heard up to 10 feet away when I moved for the first few days.

Rib fractures are common after all types of blunt trauma. They are routinely associated with a lot of pain. Most of our efforts are directed at pain relief and encouraging deep breathing and coughing even though it is extremely painful. It feels like someone is stabbing you with every cough, and sneezing . . . forgetaboutit! Many old remedies are frankly hogwash, and some may be harmful. Strapping the chest restricts respiratory movement and is potentially a real problem leading to reduced chest wall movement and potentially lung collapse. And folks in years past even rigged up a metal clawlike apparatus to place the chest wall on traction. If we limit our treatment to pain relief, encourage the patient to take big breaths, and wait about seventy-two hours, the ribs start to heal. Then, as the bones stick together, the pain improves considerably. With the most severe chest injuries, there may be bruising of the underlying lung (called a pulmonary contusion), which can complicate the care. These patients can have difficulty breathing and even end up on a ventilator for some time. Lung injuries tend to result from high-energy collisions like being fired out of a cannon into a brick wall (one of my favorite examples of a hypothetically bad trauma mechanism). A real-life example of high-energy impact is a high-speed car crash into a fixed object, like a telephone pole. A patient in this situation often sustains a multitude of injuries and is categorized jokingly as a "SLAB," which stands for "squashed like a bug." Nasty chest wounds are often accompanied by many other significant injuries requiring attention.

If a doctor has treated a man with a metal knife for a severe wound and has caused the man to die, his hands shall be cut off.

HAMMURABI'S CODE (~2000 BCE)

From 1978 to 1995, Ted Kaczynski, a.k.a. the Unabomber, killed three individuals and injured twenty-three more with his mail bombs. I was the trauma surgeon for one of his last victims, a computer scientist, wounded after one of Kaczynski's letter bombs exploded in the professor's office in 1993. The blast victim was able to run down the stairwell and over to the student health services. I am sure his appearance was quite scary for the folks in their quiet little medical clinic. He had been injured by an exploding package containing metal objects like bolts and screws. He survived severe burns, shrapnel wounds, and damage to an eye, and lost parts of one of his hands. Most life-threatening was the lung contusion from the blast, which caused him to require ventilator support. The novelty of a war-type wound in a civilian practice was given extra notoriety by association with the evil Unabomber. Therefore, I was thrust before the media daily as the chief of trauma, but I was not allowed to divulge any details due to privacy concerns even in the days before the Health Insurance Portability and Accountability Act (HIPAA). I was only a few years out of training, but I'd had some wartime experience in Desert Storm, and the basic principles of trauma management are similar in civilian and combat care.

For a number of years after the Unabomber experience, I investigated the effects of bomb blasts on the lungs. Bruising of the lung is commonly associated with serious chest wall injuries. Patients with pulmonary contusions often have difficulty breathing, require ventilator support, and can have a complicated respiratory course. This injury was often seen during World War I, but the significance was not comprehended at that time. There was no way to measure blood oxygen levels. (That would have to wait until the 1960s for clinical use.) At autopsy, WWI soldiers subjected to bomb blasts or explosions were found to have lungs filled with blood, so the lungs appeared to resemble the liver. My colleagues and

I developed an animal model of lung injury that we used to study the effects of the type of fluid for resuscitation. Unfortunately, we did not find a resuscitation method to help us avoid all the complications associated with lung injury. We now understand that blasts or explosions cause the most significant damage wherever there is an air-fluid interface. Therefore, the eardrums, the lungs, and the intestines are often injured during explosions. At this point, care for a pulmonary contusion is only supportive.

> *The greater the ignorance, the greater the dogmatism.*
> WILLIAM OSLER (1849–1919)

I saw the boy in the office, weeks after he had recovered from the trauma. He had been injured in some random collision (I think he was kicked during a soccer game), and one of my partners had removed a bleeding kidney. The parents were quite concerned about the emotional state of their sixteen-year-old son, the star athlete, now that he could "never play sports again." "Who gave you that advice?" I asked incredulously. The boy had another kidney! It turns out the family's pediatrician had been adamant that the boy could not play with only one kidney. I tried to explain to the parents that this was utter nonsense. They looked at me like I was both ignorant and frivolous. And certainly not concerned about the well-being of their son.

For decades, I subscribed to *Sports Illustrated*. I enjoyed the superb writing, the insights, and occasionally the swimsuit edition. But sometimes, even *SI* gets it wrong. On November 4, 1996, Rick Reilly, an excellent sportswriter, penned an article about a Midwestern high school senior who gave up a college scholarship and maybe an NFL career because he donated his kidney to his ailing grandmother. This story made the cover of that issue of *SI*. At the time, I was running a major trauma center in the Northeast, and my first question was, why? The odds of losing a kidney in sports (about 12 in 4,400,000) are similar to the likelihood of being struck by lightning (1 in 1,200,000).[2] And if you have only one kidney, you can wear protective body armor and be perfectly safe. The American Academy of Pediatrics, in fact, does *not* recommend prohibiting contact sports for people (boys or girls) who have a single kidney. So this young man gave up his passion and a promising football career because a physician told him something that was not based on common sense or the data. Evidence-based medicine to the rescue!

> *A specialist is a man who knows more*
> *and more about less and less.*
>
> **WILLIAM JAMES MAYO (1861–1939)**

The chief of plastic surgery at a prominent institution crashed into a pole while skiing the day before a major trauma meeting. He was flown to a trauma center, where it was determined that his facial bones had turned into dust. Typically, serious facial fractures are managed by peeling back the skin and wiring together bone fragments like a jigsaw puzzle. But this face was pulverized, so the surgeons attempted to replicate his appearance based on his driver's license photo. He never looked the same again. And that is why I carry a picture of George Clooney in my wallet . . .

After his plastic surgical residency, one of my good friends did a fellowship in craniofacial reconstruction. He found that operating all night on intoxicated individuals who had been involved in an assault or grisly car crash was exhausting. And then he learned that he could be sued after the surgery if the patient did not end up looking like Brad Pitt. This pushed my buddy to move his practice to exclusively cosmetic work in his own facility. Because of experiences such as being sued after a night of operating on complex emergencies, few plastic surgeons are interested in running to the hospital late at night. Therefore, it is particularly hard to reach subspecialty surgeons, especially plastic surgeons. No longer do hospitals require that plastic surgeons cover a certain number of days per month in the emergency center to retain hospital privileges. And the most profitable practices in plastic surgery focus on cosmetic surgery. Cosmetic surgery involves cash up front rather than fighting with insurance companies and hospitals about remuneration. Many cosmetic surgeons own their operative center where the practice hires assistants and anesthesiologists. The surgeon can reap the profitable rewards of their efforts rather than the hospital absorbing most of the dollars.

Not everyone in the plastic surgical field is ethical (or in any area of medicine, for that matter). But I am focusing on plastic surgery here. At one institution where I cared for patients, one of the senior plastic surgeons would only come in to fix facial lacerations if the patient had insurance. If the "wallet biopsy" was negative (i.e., no insurance), he would instruct the resident to perform the repair. While this is hopefully a rare phenomenon, it is concerning that some institutions allow this behavior to continue. Of all the surgical subspecialties, plastic surgery is one of the few where private practice is much more lucrative than academic practice (two to four times the income). Because it is so expensive to undergo cosmetic work in the United States, patients sometimes choose to go abroad for their surgery (medical tourism). Recently, we have treated many young women with antibiotics and drainage procedures after they've had "Brazilian butt lifts" performed in Central and South America. Buyer beware.

A man put a rifle in his mouth to commit suicide but flinched at the last second and blew off most of his face. The paramedics found his trachea bubbling in a sea of blood at the scene and put in a breathing tube. On arrival at the trauma center, both of his eyes were dangling out of his head, but he was wide awake and communicated that now he wanted to live. After many operations by the facial reconstructive surgeons, his face was partially restored (sort of).

> *I prefer to die by the decree of God rather than by the hand of man.*
>
> GUILLAUME DUPUYTREN (1777–1835)

Trauma surgeons, and members of the trauma team we work with, often must have a bit of gallows humor to help us deal with the daily doses of death and dismemberment. If we absorbed the degree of tragedy induced by injuries to both the patients and their loved ones, we would be unable to perform our life-preserving duties. Suicide attempts are kept at arm's length, so we sometimes find absurdity in how imaginative and innovative our patients can be. One evening, after a domestic dispute, a young college student was observed jumping from the twenty-second-floor balcony of a hotel and landing on the fifth-floor restaurant roof. After plummeting over 150 feet, she arrived at the ER screaming at us to let her die (which we did not). She later thanked us for saving her life after the orthopedic team repaired her hip fractures. I always kiddingly tell my kids that if they have a bad breakup with their cheating boyfriend or girlfriend, throw them *out the window, and do not jump!*

There are about forty-seven thousand suicides in the United States each year. Over half are the result of gunshot wounds. Most gunshot wound suicides occur in rural areas by middle-aged or older Caucasian men. This number of suicides by gunfire exceeds the number of homicide deaths by gunshot wounds (which typically occur among young inner-city men of color). The methods used to attempt suicide matter, as we will illustrate below.

One of the most complicated suicide attempts I treated was the patient who poured gasoline over himself, then stabbed himself in the abdomen, lacerating his duodenum (the first part of the intestine) and his vena cava (the main blood vessel to the heart), each a potentially lethal injury. He then lit himself on fire before leaping out the fourth-floor window. Naturally, he lived. But the winner for bizarre goes to the man who, on his third suicide attempt, tried to cut off his head with a big revved-up chainsaw. It bit deep into his skull, cutting into his brain, but, yes, he survived. When the neurosurgeon walked into the operating room, he quipped, "Well, at least the patient has an open mind."

But seriously, we do not know what is going through the minds of patients who attempt suicide. The rate of survival is related to the method chosen. Self-inflicted gunshot wounds (82 percent die) and hanging (61 percent) have a high fatality rate, while jumping

(31 percent) and drug overdose (1.5 percent) are much lower. We try to ascertain motivation in failed attempts at suicide and always involve psychiatric service providers to help us with all our successfully revived patients.

I had just showered after being up all night on call and was about to be filmed as part of a documentary on bloodless medicine (medical care without blood transfusions). I arrived for the taping at the conference room adjacent to the trauma resuscitation rooms in my clean white shirt and tie. My sleepless night was apparently manifesting as dark circles under my eyes. A diminutive makeup artist appeared and suggested I sit down for a touch-up. She sat behind me, applied a protective cape, and asked me to lean far back so she could work her magic. As I strained to hyperextend my neck, I began to feel dizzy. I told her I did not feel well. She repeatedly said, "Just a minute more." After a few minutes, I could not wait any longer, and I bolted up to stand. Then I passed out momentarily and went down like a falling tree. My surgical colleagues thought I had just had a heart attack, so I was loaded onto a gurney while the team prepared to perform CPR. Here I was, the director of the trauma center being rolled into our own trauma room. Kneeling on the stretcher was one of the anesthesiologists squeezing a bag to give me oxygen through a face mask and repeating, "Oh shit, oh shit." As the trauma area entry door crashed open, I tried to communicate through the mask that I was okay and pushed them all away from me. They were getting ready to put in a breathing tube and treat me like a fresh trauma patient. Initially, we thought I had had an allergic reaction to the makeup products. We ultimately figured out that this event was related to the cloth drape that the artist had wrapped tightly around my neck to protect my shirt collar before leaning me back. This cut off all the blood supply to my tiny brain.

Fortunately, I was revived and went on to complete the documentary that morning. But for some reason, in all the footage from that day, I did look kind of gray . . .

Hanging is the second-most common method of self-inflicted death in the United States after gunshot wounds. It is said that nearly two-thirds of suicide attempts by hanging are successful. Hanging represents 40 to 50 percent of all suicides worldwide but varies in prevalence from country to country. It is more common in younger age groups. Hanging suicide deaths typically occur by "suspension hanging," which involves strangulation. It only takes about 10 pounds of pressure on the carotid arteries in the neck to occlude them, and one becomes unconscious in seconds, but death is said to occur in about four minutes. By contrast, in executions by "drop hanging," the individual is dropped about 5 to 6 feet to snap the neck and injure the spinal cord. This is thought to be a more "humane" form of execution by hanging. The hanging victims we see in the trauma center are typically unsuccessful suicide attempts, and our job is to rule out associated injury to the bones and soft tissues of the neck and to manage any resulting brain injury from the transient lack of oxygen.

> *The natural force within each of us is that greatest healer of all.*
>
> HIPPOCRATES (460–377 BCE)

A young high school soccer player was out at a party with his friends, and things got rowdy. He was separated from his friends when someone pulled out a handgun and everyone scattered. As he ran away from the shooter,

*he was struck in the back of the knee, and the bullet cut through his pop-
liteal artery (the blood vessel to the lower leg). He was alone in the street
for hours before someone picked him up and brought him to the trauma
center. The artery was repaired immediately, but the delay was too much
for his lower leg muscles and nerves, which were irreversibly damaged.
He had developed compartment syndrome and was left with permanent
foot drop (he would never be able to pull his toes off the ground). Just like
that, his athletic days were over.*

I have reviewed several cases where a patient developed severe
extremity pain after an injury and later lost a limb or significant
leg function due to a delay in diagnosis of compartment syndrome.
Acute compartment syndrome results from increased pressures in
a muscle compartment of an extremity, classically the lower leg,
leading to a reduction in blood flow. The tissues receive inadequate
oxygen and die. A good example is when a car bumper strikes a
pedestrian's leg, breaking the bone and bruising the surrounding
tissues. If there is sufficient swelling from the injury, pressures in
the space around the fractured bone will rise and may exceed pressures in the veins. This leads to more swelling and more significant
pressures surpassing arterial pressures (so blood flow stops). The
first sign of compartment syndrome is often tingling in the foot,
followed by numbness. Then we see pain that can rise to an
extremely severe level. When the syndrome is quite advanced, the
leg muscles feel rock-hard. The key to preventing tissue loss and
permanent nerve damage is quickly recognizing the potential
problem and opening the space around the muscle (called a fasci-
otomy). This requires some experience and judgment. Waiting
even a few extra hours can have severe consequences.

The young man was sent quickly to the operating room to repair his severely broken ankle sustained during a hard tackle in a soccer game. After surgery, he was loaded into the back seat of a car for a long drive home. During the trip, he complained of severe pain in his leg. His parents stopped at an emergency room, where the physicians expressed concern about the severity of his pain. The doctors arranged to fly him to the nearest trauma center. The orthopedist at the trauma center was called but declined to come to the hospital, feeling that this was normal postoperative pain. During the night, the patient's pain could not be controlled with the usual medications. Early the following day, the patient underwent exploratory surgery and was found to have acute compartment syndrome. Fortunately, he did not lose his leg.

A man is as old as his arteries.

Thomas Sydenham (1624–1689)

The marine had returned home after his second tour in Iraq. He went to the gun shop to get a new laser sight for the Glock handgun that he had just received as a gift. That weapon lacks a separate safety mechanism and is fired when enough force is applied to the trigger. He was trying to attach the new part to his gun in the parking lot when it discharged and blew a hole in his leg, lacerating his popliteal artery (which carries the blood supply to the leg below the knee). Realizing that he was bleeding actively, he wisely wrapped his belt around his mid-thigh and cinched it up like a tourniquet. That simple act helped save his leg and his life.

For many years, tourniquets had a bad reputation. I am sure that their misuse was associated with limb loss in the past. But the Israeli military rejuvenated the use of this device, proving that it could save limbs and lives with short-term, appropriate use. Subsequently, the US Department of Defense improved upon tourniquets, making them easier to apply and with a single hand, no less. Surgeons' experience of caring for soldiers in Iraq and Afghanistan has been quite positive regarding tourniquets. Tourniquets do not cause damage but rather prevent exsanguination (bleeding out all of one's blood volume) and limb loss.

The patient mentioned above underwent repair of his injured artery that evening, but first we placed something called a vascular shunt. It is a piece of plastic tubing inserted inside the artery to permit blood flow—in this case, to the lower leg. This process of flow restoration with a shunt is immediate, while it often takes some time (minutes to hours) to reconnect an artery. If the patient requires other procedures simultaneously, like having broken bones repaired, shunts allow time to address other issues. This is particularly valuable in a war zone, where patients may need to be stabilized before being transferred to a higher-level facility. If the patient is too unstable to withstand the time it takes to do this very technical procedure, the shunt buys time. Likewise, if the operative team lacks a surgeon capable of performing a vascular anastomosis (connecting the two ends of the blood vessel, often using graft material), a shunt can be inserted and will allow hours of blood flow while the patient awaits transfer to another facility. The use of shunts has helped save many limbs. It turns out that every hour's delay in restoring blood flow dramatically increases the risk of amputation.

After you have been up all night operating, it is hard to generate enthusiasm to do meticulous vascular surgery. If vascular work is not done precisely, blood does not flow, and you must refashion the entire connection between the ends of the blood vessels. I remember one tough night when we were in the OR for twelve hours straight with multiple cases, including more than one that required vascular anastomosis. At about 6:30 a.m., thirty minutes before the next team was to appear, a man arrived with a gunshot wound to the pelvis. We explored his abdomen and groin area and found an injury to the femoral artery (the major blood vessel to the leg) right under the inguinal ligament. As mentioned earlier regarding a similar injury, think of the scene in the movie Black Hawk Down, *in which an army ranger died from bleeding after a bullet wound to the groin. The hard part of dealing with this injury is gaining control of the bleeding. The bullet had destroyed a couple of inches of the blood vessel, so we prepared to sew in a piece of graft tubing, which is routine for vascular injuries in medium-sized blood vessels. The chief resident and I repeatedly cut the plastic graft material in an attempt to fashion the appropriate shape but could not get it exactly right. We were a bit bleary-eyed at that time. Finally, I said to my assistant, "Do you even want to finish this case?" "Not really," he responded. So we called in the fresh new team, who were ecstatic to help. They got to perform the critical part of the operation, with everything all exposed and ready to go. Having done all the heavy lifting for the next team, we headed to the donut shop for a cup of coffee and a chocolate donut and continued with our day.*

> *The keen clinician, as he grows in experience, becomes more and more valuable as age advances.*
>
> WILLIAM J. MAYO (1861–1939)

After a grueling thirty hours in the hospital, I had just returned home when my phone rang. "Do you know Dave?" a paramedic asked me from the scene of an accident. Dave, the surgical resident working in our animal physiology laboratory, had a love for high-performance Italian motorcycles. He had crashed his motorbike and managed to dislocate his ankle so that his foot was twisted over onto the side of his leg. Dave asked them to call me immediately, and I could hear him yelling in pain in the background. I directed the medic to head to the trauma center and jumped in my car to drive back to the hospital. Amazingly, Dave's ankle was able to be relocated by our orthopedists while Dave was under anesthesia, and he had no broken bones or destroyed ligaments. Fortunately, it is rare for our friends and family to have injuries, but we certainly hear about it and try to help ensure optimal care. Dave went on to become an Ironman triathlete, special forces surgeon, and trauma surgeon at a major teaching hospital in Boston. He even treated some of the Boston Marathon bombing victims after finishing the race himself.

The scary joint dislocations are not fingers, shoulders, or even ankles, but hips and, most dreaded, knees. We see occasional hip dislocations, primarily in unbelted passengers who slide forward and compress their knee on the dash in high-speed head-on car crashes. This injury is pretty obvious, as the affected leg is shortened and immobile, with great hip pain on manipulation. These are emergencies, as failure to relocate the dislocated hip can lead to necrosis of the head of the femur. Once the hip is back in place, blood flow is restored to the bone, and the patient usually avoids a hip replacement.

Knee dislocations are much more subtle and dangerous than hip dislocations and are challenging to diagnose. Often, they present after significant trauma as just a swollen knee related to blood in the knee joint. The knee can dislocate and then return to the normal position (this is called subluxation), with disruption of the stabilizing ligaments of the knee. While this is problematic because it may require the repair of damaged cartilage or ligaments, the real danger is that the blood supply to the lower leg can be disrupted. The injury can be missed initially, as the patient can have normal pulses. Failure to diagnose an arterial injury could lead to a decrease in blood flow to the lower leg and even loss of the leg. Therefore, every major trauma victim with a swollen knee is considered to have had a dislocation and undergoes an evaluation of the blood vessels in the leg.

> *Sports teach you how to be quick.*
> *Injuries teach you how to slow down.*
>
> YAO MING (1980–)

During one of my college basketball tournaments, a good athlete on the opposing team was playing entirely out of control. I usually would not say anything, but this guy was dangerous. As we ran down the court, I told him, "Dude, you are going to hurt someone. Chill." But he did not. A few plays later, as our 6-foot-8-inch power forward grabbed a rebound, this hyped-up guy jumped up and bounced off the rebounder's back and fell into my face. His forehead smashed into my nose, crushing it into pieces. My already naturally misshapen schnozzle was now bent over almost to my ear. As blood spurted out of my face, I sat down while the fast break took off down the court behind me. The worst part of this experience was that I had to have my nose rebuilt the next day and miss a great outdoor rock concert. The best part was I had a lovely picture of my bent beak to send to my mom for Mother's Day, with me looking like the Penguin after getting punched by Batman.

I was playing in a pickup basketball game during my residency years with some folks who did not understand the game. Rather than play defense, one guy decided to just knock me down. As I hit the asphalt, my wrist immediately began to hurt. I was aware that I may have had a significant injury, one that would require immobilization of my wrist in a cast, and so on. I naturally ignored it for two weeks. Finally, unable to turn a doorknob, I got an X-ray that confirmed that I had a scaphoid fracture. This bone in the wrist is often injured when a person falls on their outstretched hand. Unfortunately, these bones often do not heal on their own. This injury requires prolonged immobilization in a cast for about six weeks. And still, nearly half of the folks do not heal their injuries and surgery is needed. As I was a senior surgical resident at the time, I elected to cut off my cast after a couple of weeks so that I could operate. Fortunately, my wrist healed. But I do not advise this boneheaded maneuver at all.

A surgeon, an internist, and a pathologist went duck hunting. The first person up was the internist. There was rustling in the bushes, and up flew a duck. The internist said, pointing his weapon, "Looks like a duck, but might be a hawk or an eagle" as the duck flew off. Next up was the surgeon. As the bird rose in the air, the surgeon fired his shotgun. Down came the fowl. "Why don't you tell me if that is a duck," the surgeon directed the pathologist.

ANONYMOUS

When my nine-year-old daughter, Elizabeth, hurt her shoulder after being thrown in jujitsu, she was convinced she needed an X-ray. I told her we would ice the area and wait till the morning, as there was no deformity and minimal tenderness. "No," she said, "it popped, and I need an

X-ray." Daddy prevailed. The next morning, she woke screaming in pain,
now with an obvious deformity from her broken clavicle. "You are the
worst trauma surgeon in the world," she informed me. Hope not.

The common adage in my family was that you would not get
much attention for an injury unless you were bleeding to death. A
trauma surgeon's kids do have to grow up in a strange environment. On the one hand, if they have an injury and are taken to the
trauma center, the Red Sea parts. Both the chief of plastic surgery
and the chief of oral surgery are there to immediately sew up what
turned out to be a tiny 1-inch chin laceration. (This happened
with my daughter when she was in nursery school.) The wife of
one of my partners had bad abdominal pain one day. At the trauma
center, we did multiple imaging studies, the gynecologist and the
surgeon on call saw her, and she underwent an appendectomy and
was moved to the recovery room. All in about an hour. This is
usually a process that would take six to eight hours. On the other
hand, my kids would say that they had to be dying to get any
medical attention from their parents (especially me). My son was
playing soccer in the backyard barefoot and sliced open his foot.
As I walked calmly from the house to check out his injury, he
yelled, "Why aren't you freaking out?" Over a little bit of blood?

But there are times when having a surgeon around is valuable.
When my son was a little over a year old, he was a complete terror.
We used to say, "It was a good day . . . less than fifty near-death
experiences." One day, as I walked into the house from work, I
heard a scream: "Sam's not breathing!" I ran to the kitchen where
my wife had our boy upside down and was beating him like a rug.
He had climbed up on the kitchen table and aspirated a handful

of peanuts. Now he was blue, not breathing, and about to die. I grabbed his ankles and gave him three hard back claps while looking for the block of kitchen knives. "Please don't make me trach my baby boy," I prayed. Fortunately, out came a gush of peanuts, and he started to breathe. Clearly, he was brain-damaged, as he went on to become an attorney. (Kidding!!!)

I should insert here that the Heimlich maneuver (now referred to as abdominal thrusts) is no longer recommended as the initial management of choking by the Red Cross. Instead, it now recommends five back blows first. Abdominal thrusts are potentially dangerous and are not as effective as the back clap.

If anyone should doubt whether the electrical matter passes through the substance of bodies, or only over along their surfaces, a shock from an electrified large glass jar, taken through his own body, will probably convince him.

BENJAMIN FRANKLIN (1706–1790)

I was power washing off the dock at a vacation home in the Florida Keys around dusk. No one was at the house but me. As the sun dropped below the horizon, I needed more illumination from the lamps on the boat lift to see what I was doing. I went inside the porch and flipped on the light switch, but nothing happened. I figured the bulb was out. I returned to the dock and was standing in a puddle of water when my sleeve must have touched a light pole with an electrical short, and my entire body started to jerk rhythmically. As the current passed through my body, I realized that I was receiving an electrical shock and was about to be electrocuted (that is when you die from electrical injury). Before I could pass out, I threw myself up and backward, breaking the connection.

I landed on my back several feet away with a thud, dazed and tingling.
Better than being found days later as a crispy critter.

In the United States, there are about one thousand deaths per year because of electrical injuries. Approximately four hundred are due to high-voltage electrical injuries, and lightning kills about fifty, leaving around 350 dying from lower-voltage injuries. There are also at least thirty thousand shock incidents per year that are non-fatal. Around 5 percent of all burn unit admissions in the United States occur because of electrical injuries, and about 20 percent of these occur in children (kids chew through a lot of electrical cords).[3]

Lightning is particularly fascinating because it is a direct current, so the injuries are different from when a power line zaps someone. Lightning can involve a large amount of current, which is more important than the voltage applied. Therefore, it can induce more damage. According to the CDC, the odds of being struck by lightning are about one in a million each year, but there are certainly higher-risk areas (the highest incidence rate in the United States is in Florida). Of the folks who die from lightning strikes each year in the United States, 85 percent are men. One-third of lightning strikes, surprisingly, occur in individuals who remain indoors. Two-thirds of lightning injuries happen between noon and 6 p.m.

The scary thing about electrical injuries is that the external signs of damage may be minimal, but the amount of tissue scorched by the passage of current can be extensive. The heart can beat abnormally, but patients in cardiac arrest can often be zapped back, even from a complete standstill. Therefore, patients exposed to electrical injuries are treated a bit differently from the usual burn patient. They are closely monitored for cardiac abnormalities and evidence of muscle tissue damage where the current passed through the patient. Because of improved safety measures, we do not see as many workplace electrical injuries today as in years past.

> *The surgical investigator must be a bridge tender,*
> *channeling knowledge from biological science to*
> *the patient's bedside and back again.*
>
> FRANCIS D. MOORE (1913–2001)

A two-year-old boy was brought in extremis (near death) to the trauma center covered with deep-appearing dog bites. His grandmother's two pit bulls had attacked him. Grandma had tried to get the dogs off the child by stabbing them, and they were subsequently shot by the police. The little boy had bled severely, and we could not resuscitate him. Grandma was injured but survived. The trauma service was so disturbed that the trauma fellow and I decided to research dog bites as a line of investigation.

This section is challenging for me to write as I am the ultimate dog lover and have had many wonderful dogs. However, about one million Americans seek medical attention for dog bites each year. Of this number, only approximately thirty thousand patients require surgery for severe bites, and about twenty-five die from bites. While breeds such as cocker spaniels top the list most years of dogs that bite, they do not do much damage. There are, however, several breeds of dogs that can cause severe damage when they attack. Foremost on that list are pit bulls (half of all catastrophic dog bites) and rottweilers (25 percent of severe bites). The term "pit bull" actually includes four breeds: the American Pit Bull Terrier, the American Staffordshire Terrier, the Staffordshire Bull Terrier, and the American Bully. And the term is often applied to mixed breeds that have a component of the Bull Terrier.

If we benchmark the risk of catastrophic dog bites to the Labrador retriever (the most common dog breed), the risk of being maimed by a German shepherd is only four times that of a Lab; the risk of being maimed by a rottweiler is sixty-six times that of a Lab. More disturbing, the odds of death or dismemberment from a pit bull attack are twenty-five hundred times that of a Labrador. There are historical reasons why pit bulls can be ferocious. These dogs were bred in the twelfth century to attack bulls and other dogs. They were chosen because they show no sign of impending attack (meaning that they do not typically snarl, growl, or show their teeth) and are relentless and quite strong for their weight. Pit bulls can certainly induce catastrophic damage.[4]

In around 2010, when I was researching an article on dog bites, I had the opportunity to talk to a CDC director who was an expert on this subject. I suggested that perhaps we should outlaw pit bulls nationally as they did in Denver and Toronto. I was informed that I had it completely wrong. The CDC expert said that they had studied this and found that if we made pit bulls illegal, those owners would just buy a wolf. But an excellent solution was unveiled in Barcelona, Spain, and the surrounding region. Officials in this area enforced an ordinance requiring owners of about fourteen higher-risk dog breeds to take a safety course, follow specific regulations, and carry insurance. These regulations led to a 50 percent reduction in severe dog attacks that was sustained for more than a decade. Certainly, this supports the concept that responsible ownership of high-risk dog breeds can dramatically limit the likelihood of injury.

In most regions of the United States, dogs are considered safe until they bite someone—the "one-bite rule." From that point, they are regarded as a risk to the populace (think a loaded gun), and the owner is legally responsible if any damage occurs from subsequent biting events. Of course, this typically leads to the dog being euthanized. National Public Radio once interviewed me and my colleague on a Maryland law categorizing pit bulls as biting dogs without requiring prior injury. They asked me my opinion on outlawing pit bulls, and I reiterated the need for regulations like those in Barcelona. Strangely, no one would question special rules for owners of exotic predators like mountain lions, as they are not domesticated. But pit bulls (and other high-risk dogs) are treated like poodles in terms of community safety, which can lead to severe injuries if the owners are reckless.

> *Dogs never bite me—just humans.*
> MARILYN MONROE (1926–1962)

As an intern on the plastic surgery service, I helped cover the emergency room for one of the busier county hospitals in the United States. I was constantly calling my senior, the plastic surgery fellow, at home with crazy stories that I invented to amuse him. But one night, a patient arrived who had filleted the back of his thumb with a kitchen knife and injured the extensor tendon. This is the tendon that allows you to lift your thumb. Usually, these tendons are repaired semi-electively, but in this case, the man was a flamenco guitarist who had stopped in our city on the way to Los Angeles for a recording session. After convincing my chief that this was not a fabrication, he drove in, and we repaired the man's injury as an emergency. Covering the hand service, I would often see men with huge swollen hands who needed emergency operations. They had typically struck someone in the teeth during a fight at a drinking establishment the night prior and sustained "human bites."

When most people think of bites by humans, they visualize a little kid nibbling on another little kid. Or Mike Tyson munching on Evander Holyfield's ear in a heavyweight boxing match. But the usual human "bite" that we see in the trauma center occurs after one person punches another person in the mouth. That is how we refer to this particular injury, which is obviously not an intentional bite (rarely do we see someone who has been gnawed on by another person). When someone is hit in the mouth, their teeth can break the assailant's skin, usually over the knuckles, and inoculate the tissues with the infectious organisms that live in our mouths. The primary culprit is a bacteria called *Eikenella corrodens*, which is quite virulent (meaning an aggressive organism that spreads rapidly). Typically, someone arrives late in the morning after they sober up. They were in a bar fight the prior evening. Now they have a massive swollen hand and no recollection of any injury. These folks require an operation to wash out the area of injury and repair any underlying damage. And large doses of antibiotics. Failure to seek and receive immediate treatment for these human "bites" can have dire consequences for hand function. Human bites are more dangerous than dog or cat bites from an infection standpoint. Usually, animal bites only require irrigation and wound care in the ER, with some antibiotic pills. Rarely do they cause significant infections requiring admission, as human bites do.

Of course, people are not concerned about rabies from a human bite. Rabies is always a concern, however, after bites from animals. According to the CDC, about five thousand cases of rabies in animals are reported annually in the United States. Most of these (over 90 percent) occur from wildlife. Before 1960, most cases were found in domestic animals, like dogs. Since that time, the rabies reservoir has been found in bats, raccoons, skunks, and foxes. Only about one human dies from rabies in the United States per year, which is remarkably decreased from the early twentieth century, when over one hundred deaths yearly were recorded. The CDC attributes this decline to several factors: successful pet vaccination, animal control programs, public health surveillance, testing, and the availability of post-exposure prophylaxis for rabies.

When spider webs unite, they can tie up a lion.

Ethiopian proverb

I was moving across the country with the entire family and our Labrador, Rosebud, heading to my new job as a trauma center director in Florida. Because of Rosebud, we had a limited selection of lodging. While Rosebud was truly the best dog ever, when we attempted to bring her into the pet-permitted motel in rural Georgia, she uncharacteristically hit the brakes and would not set one paw in the room. It must have been teeming with fleas or something. I should have listened to Rosebud . . .

We had to leave the dog in the car, and I got up every hour or two all night to take Rosebud for a walk and give her some water, as it was incredibly hot and humid. After my 6 a.m. dog walk, I was in the bathroom, having just washed my hands in the dark, when I felt extreme pain in my ring finger. I flipped on the lights but could not see what had chomped on me. That day, we drove the remaining distance into Florida but had to stop the car at my new trauma center to have my ring cut off, as my finger was swelling massively. We surmised that a black widow spider had attacked me. Thank you, Georgia.

I grew up in the San Francisco Bay Area of Northern California, not that far from the black widow capital of the world, Davis, California. I was always a bit careful around spiders. We all know that these critters are good for the environment, but they can be a little bit creepy. Anyway, I had never had a severe spider bite until my trip through Georgia, and there are not a lot of insects that can cause the kind of reaction that I had. In addition to losing my wedding band, I had to get a steroid injection and antibiotics. And part of my finger sloughed off. Both black widow and brown recluse spiders produce dangerous venoms and represent the most hazardous spiders in North America. And their bites, from personal experience, hurt like the devil.

> *Indeed, above all else, a wound must be made clean.*
> THEODORIC (1205–1296)

The man arrived at the ER with an arm cast that reeked to high heaven. It had been in place for over a year, during which he had not bothered to return to the hospital for follow-up. He was mentally unbalanced, homeless, and living in the wild. He had decided to visit us because friends complained that worms were climbing out of the end of his cast. We removed the plaster from his wrist to reveal an open wound where the bones were not healed and maggots were having a picnic. Now he would need an extended hospitalization to clean up the wound, and the bone would need to be stabilized with an external fixator (a set of metal rods that go through the skin to align the bones). In the healthcare community, we are accustomed to dealing with this type of patient, as we have many neglected, poverty-stricken individuals that we see at the safety-net hospitals. We try to treat them the same as anyone else, but their care can be challenging.

Many therapies have stood the test of time. In the 1970s, a study from North Africa looked at complicated infected wounds that were treated with either the modern methods of antibiotics, wound debridement, and wound dressings (our standard Western treatment) or the application of honey alone. There were no differences in outcomes. Honey has antibacterial and barrier characteristics, but most of us in the West continue to reserve honey for our hot cross buns.

Maggots are still used to treat complicated chronic wounds. Some companies make "medicinal maggots," which are fly larvae (they are acquired from a medical supply facility). These are applied to chronic wounds, usually for about forty-eight hours, under a nylon stocking (to minimize escape). Leaving the maggots in place for too long can permit them to mature into blowflies that will circulate throughout hospital rooms. This "biosurgery" can be quite effective. It is typically reserved for wounds for which operative debridement would be treacherous, like when dead tissue is overlying an important ligament or nerve. The maggots prioritize the consumption of dead tissue, but if they are left for long enough, they will eat normal tissue. Health insurance does cover this treatment, and it is used at the discretion of the clinician. While there are no large trials comparing biosurgery with conventional operative debridement, there is quite a bit of clinical experience. But maggots do seem to work for specific chronic wound conditions. One of my partners employed maggot therapy for many complicated wounds that no one else wanted to treat. He stopped using biosurgery, however, when the hospital staff started referring to him as the "Maggot Doctor."

> *"Though the doctors treated him . . .*
> *he nevertheless recovered."*
>
> LEO TOLSTOY (1828–1910)

We got a call from a cruise ship off the Bahamas requesting the transport of an injured passenger. We received many of these calls as one of the leading trauma centers serving the Caribbean. Helicopter transport arrived with a young woman who had a severely injured pelvis. On their honeymoon, the frisky couple had gotten a bit imaginative on the upper-deck balcony during an act of passion. The new bride had spilled over the railing, falling a considerable distance to the boat deck. Fortunately, she had not sustained a head injury, and our orthopedic surgeons could put our little acrobat together again.

One of my colleagues worked on a huge cruise ship as the ship doctor for a while. He subsequently wrote a TV script about the "sick bay" as a unique place on board where the three thousand guests and the two thousand support crew converge and were all medically treated. The ship's doctor is rarely a surgeon, so some imaginative and creative variations in injury management must be provided. Certainly, no physician can be an expert in all areas of medicine. From a trauma perspective, there is always the usual "gravity and dumbass," but there are also injuries generated by violence between crew members and, more rarely, passengers. In one instance, a crew member was airlifted to us after another worker slit his throat open when a love triangle went awry. Someone had sewn the skin closed over a gaping hole in the trachea, still bleeding and leaking air under the skin on the patient's arrival. Another patient arrived from a cruise in a coma from severe renal failure. He had been bitten by a poisonous snake while rafting as part of a cruise ship excursion. Both of these patients survived, barely.

Notably, these ships dock at ports on islands where there may be little in the way of emergency medical support. I was once speaking at a symposium on a large, popular Caribbean island. A government minister asked me to discuss designing a prehospital provider support (EMTs and paramedics) for the area between the two most-frequented vacation destination cities. These tourist areas are where cruise ships disembark scores of passengers to frolic in the waves. Around 2017, the government of this particular island provided zero emergency medical support for at least part of the island. I had visited some of the island's hospitals, which were nicely equipped with well-trained personnel, but there was simply no ambulance network to take a person to the trauma centers. It now appears that EMS services are available in the population centers of the island.

7

MANAGING THE PUBLIC

As I esteem the honours which have been conferred upon me,
I regard all worldly distinctions as nothing in comparison with
the hope that I may have been the means of reducing in some
degree the sum of human misery.
JOSEPH LISTER (1827–1912)

I sat down to a family meeting with a middle-aged woman whose husband had sustained a significant head and chest injury and some major extremity fractures in a high-speed car crash. The bedside ICU nurse and surgical resident joined us in a private setting. The wife stressed that this man was her entire life, and she loved him so much. We reported that he was doing quite well and was waking up and weaning off the ventilator. The woman suggested that she would happily give blood or even donate a kidney if we could assure her that he would survive. I informed her that her husband still needed some orthopedic repair of his broken legs, but we expected him to do well. I added that the woman in the car with him was also improving after some significant injuries. Like CGI in a sci-fi movie, the wife morphed in attitude and physical appearance from a sweet middle-aged woman to an alien monster as she snarled, "What woman was in the car with him?" Without waiting for a reply, she exploded. "Turn off the ventilator. Pull the plug now!" she yelled. And she was not kidding. We, of course, refused to euthanize "the love of her life." The two patients were discharged alive and well.

Trauma surgeons, particularly in our roles as directors of a surgical intensive care unit, must frequently chat with families of critically ill patients after they have sustained injuries. Unlike surgeons who develop relationships with patients and their family members during the planning of elective surgical procedures (think a kidney transplant recipient), we are thrust on families without their consent. When you roll your car, you cannot select who will care for you—it is whoever is on call at the trauma center. Therefore, we are not regarded as trusted providers but rather strangers, informing the family members of the catastrophic nature of injuries sustained by their loved ones. The responses of kin are naturally unpredictable. Patients typically have not discussed their desires for heroic medical care with their kin, so families are often at a loss regarding what the critically ill person would want. Guilt-plagued relatives have different opinions, and family dynamics often lead to struggles over control of final decisions. Most of us would rather deal with discovering the hidden injuries sustained by the patients than negotiate with family members and their underlying pathology. And the adage is true that all families (including my own) are dysfunctional in their own unique way.

Note, it is a *right* of all citizens to be healthy in the rest of the developed world, not a *privilege*. In the United States, we have no *right* to be healthy; rather, it is a *privilege*. But ironically, in the United States, no one can tell a family it is time to cease caring for their terminally ill relative. Therefore, we spend fantastic sums of money sustaining the lives of dying individuals. And a considerable proportion of the national healthcare budget is expended in the last months of patients' lives. Giving futile care is wasteful—consuming precious ICU beds and tying up ICU nursing staff—and frustrating for the caretakers. Realize that when the ICU is jammed with dying individuals with no likelihood of survival, other patients who would benefit from the ICU level of care are stuck in the emergency room or the recovery room, often for days. And there is good data that ER overcrowding and delayed access to ICU care lead to increases in death and complications in patients locked in a holding pattern.[1] As there are often no financial consequences in the United States to the patient (taxpayers are saddled with the huge bill), the family members feel no pressure to move forward quickly with a decision. For an occasional patient, this would not be a significant problem. But there are often many patients for whom care is futile in the surgical ICU, so it can be very trying for the ICU team.

A layperson might respond, how do we know when care is futile? Are we, the critical care team, too quick to write off family members because they are old/difficult/taking up resources? It is hard to trust the doctors' assessment that care is futile. Everyone has a story about a parent or grandparent who died by "medical error" (including me). And families focus on "miraculous recoveries" that they hear about by word of mouth. Let me respond to this by saying that I understand the family's concerns and can empathize.

Recognize that not every bad patient outcome is the fault of the healthcare providers. I remember an angry family blaming the ICU team because their father was dying. The man had advanced alcoholic cirrhosis of the liver, metastatic cancer of the pancreas, and severe heart failure. All three conditions were individually in the terminal stages. But it was somehow the fault of the hospital and the group of individuals caring for him that he was doing so poorly.

We have a process whereby we regularly organize family meetings to include key family decision-makers, the ICU staff (physician assistants, nurses, doctors), and social workers. At times we include clergy members. This process takes a lot of time and effort. Unfortunately, many families have already decided that the critical care team members are somehow the enemy and that we are failing to do everything we can for their loved ones. Remember, the patients are in the ICU (certainly the surgical ICU) because of injuries they sustained or due to complications resulting from the care of a surgeon or a provider, not a member of the ICU team. The patient's underlying medical condition or disease process may have led them to become critically ill. Or it may be a poor decision to operate or a technical error during surgery that resulted in the patient's critical illness. But we in the ICU are the face of care at that point. And we certainly aim to advise the family members with the best data we have available as to the likely outcome and help them do what the patient would have wanted.

Here is a recent example of what we deal with daily. A ninety-year-old patient arrived at the ER after suffering a stroke. After the appropriate, evidence-based medical therapy to dissolve his clot, he had a massive brain bleed, a devastating complication and a known risk of this treatment. He underwent emergency brain surgery to evacuate a large amount of blood and then remained in a coma. The neurologist and neurosurgeon declared that there was no hope for recovery after an appropriate observation period of a week. We explained to the family that we had two options: a tracheostomy for long-term respiratory support with a feeding tube or withdrawal of care. The family stated that the patient had previously made it clear he would never want to be maintained in a persistent vegetative state. But they just could not agree to the withdrawal of care. We could not move him out of the ICU or out of the hospital without the procedures (tracheostomy and feeding tube). So he remained in the ICU for another two weeks until finally, after many more meetings, the family decided to withdraw care. Imagine dealing with three or four patients in the ICU like this every day. The ICU director and the entire ICU team often feel extremely frustrated by the agonizingly slow pace of the decision-making process. We understand that this is a unique and personal catastrophe for the family members, but we have all seen this patient/family scenario played out many times.

We clinicians do not always help our cause in the "trust Olympics," meaning that we are working mightily to gain the confidence of the family members. At one institution, a young man sustained a gunshot wound to his head while playing with a weapon he thought was not loaded. The bullet went across his brain and did devastating damage. He had brain matter leaking out of the side of his head. His aunt was a police detective who'd previously had positive experiences at the hospital. This was a good thing. We declared him brain dead with several tests, and the organ donor network evaluated him. In an extreme outlier, a neurologist who had not discussed the case with the ICU team ran out to tell the family that he had detected some unexplainable reflex twitch and therefore thought the patient was not brain dead.

Really. The boy was gone. Fortunately, his family did not react negatively. Imagine if they went to the papers with "Brain dead patient deemed alive." We would have had every patient's family whose loved one had been declared brain dead over the past decades suing the hospital for wrongful death.

The moral of the story is that we critical care clinicians are constantly striving to build trust with the families of our catastrophically ill or injured patients. As each family is a unique mystery, there are naturally some significant barriers to securing people's confidence when it comes to making life-and-death decisions.

Father Knows Best
TV SERIES FROM 1954 TO 1960

From 1969 to 1976, a popular TV show called *Marcus Welby, M.D.* featured a sincere, brilliant general practitioner in Southern California. My father was written up in the American Academy of Family Physicians in the late 1970s, in an article called "A Day in the Life of a Real Marcus Welby M.D." And he was the kind of caring, organized individual that everyone would want to have as their doctor. At Herrick Memorial Hospital in Berkeley, California, where he would rise to the position of chairman of the board of directors, he was very highly regarded. I learned this in an unusual way. While in college, I got a job as a ward clerk in that hospital's emergency room. I heard how the nursing and medical staff felt about my dad. The satisfaction that he received while taking care of his patients and everyone's respect for him convinced me to choose a career in medicine.

When I was in medical school, my father sent me a several-page handwritten account of a long clinical case each week featuring his latest medical mystery. He had a large practice in the San Francisco Bay Area, where I grew up in the '60s—a crazy time. He had done a rotating internship, followed by a year of internal medicine and then another year as a surgical resident. A three-year training period in the days when most family practitioners just did an internship was an anomaly. This undoubtedly informed his decisions when he helped set up family practice residencies in California later in his career. He would always participate in his patients' surgeries, assisting in the more significant cases. He felt it allowed him to maintain quality control and help with intraoperative decision-making. Knowing what the patient and their family desire is critical during surgery. And my dad sometimes had the perspective of five generations within a single family.

I worked in my father's office a few times as a medical secretary training new staff. I would make him crazy, wanting more to do. My mother worked as his assistant and bookkeeper in the mornings for decades after she recovered from a severe illness. They had the same nurse, Dolly, in the office for more than twenty years. Dolly used to gab with all the patients for hours, driving my father nuts. But my mother would remind my dad that most of his patients came to chat with Dolly as well as their doctor and that this was a key aspect of their wellness family. Sometimes a new patient would see my parents having lunch together and gossip to Dolly. She never gave away the doctor's secret that he was having a secret rendezvous . . . with his wife. When he was sixty-nine, he retired, not because of changes in medical care or reimbursement (as he loved taking care of his patients) but to spend more time with my mother, whom he adored.

> *I hope my surgeon is a Republican.*
> Ronald Reagan (1911–2004)

It was Valentine's Day, and I saw a billboard for a flower shop with a familiar name. I had treated the owner, who had sustained a severe liver and kidney injury after a high-speed car crash. She was the matriarch of a large family with whom I had spent a lot of time during her very rocky hospital course. The florist shop was packed with maybe fifty men doing last-minute purchasing of flowers for their honeys. As I walked into the establishment, I was engulfed by the entire family, including the former patient, who ran over to me to give me big hugs. They then put together a massive bouquet (worthy of a Kentucky Derby winner). I insisted on paying something for this immense arrangement. "For you, thirty-five dollars," they said cheerily for what was undoubtedly hundreds of dollars' worth of gorgeous blooms. The next man in line was asked what he would like to order. Mirroring the famous scene from When Harry Met Sally, *he said, "I'll have what he's having." Fat chance.*

Doctors always say it is a terrible idea to be treated as a very important person. While the rich and famous pay for top treatment and spare no expense, they often get worse rather than better hospital care. One of the problems is that other physicians (typically specialists), who may or may not be competent, show up and try to direct care. One of my residents told me about caring for a very famous musician who arrived at an outlying hospital with a gastrointestinal surgical emergency. His cardiologist insisted on directing patient care himself, and the delay in management led to the death of the patient. Every physician becomes an expert in your condition if you are a VIP. In New York City, everyone wants to be seen by their "Big Docta." So those that actually know what they are doing can be largely ignored.

In the ICU, for example, patient management requires a quarterback (typically the intensivist and the ICU team) to integrate the often-competing interests of the consultants. A kidney specialist may recommend increasing fluids to improve kidney function, while a cardiologist may want to restrict fluids because of concerns about fluid overload stressing the heart. The ICU team must collaborate with everyone while effectively delivering optimal care to the patient. And optimal care is often a moving target as the patient's needs change. Family members (particularly if they happen to be physicians or nurses) are usually adamant about what is best for the patient, usually after consulting with "Dr. Google." This represents another obstacle to delivering optimal care. The issue for family members is they fear that medical error is common, which it is. According to the World Health Organization (WHO), in high-income countries, it is estimated that one in every ten patients is harmed while receiving hospital care.[2]

The harm can be caused by various adverse events, with 50 percent of them being preventable. Some investigators claim that medical errors in the United States are underreported and may represent the third-leading cause of death. The total loss in the United States has been estimated at more than 250,000 deaths per year (or 10 percent of all deaths). A medical error (forgetting to continue to supply essential medication to someone chronically on steroids for nearly sixty years) led to my mother's demise. This occurred even though my father and I were both physicians, hovering at her bedside. Fortunately, most medical errors are not lethal, and hospitals are working diligently to maximize the safety and effectiveness of care.

I would be remiss if I did not mention the occasional benefits of dealing with very important people. Some years ago, our trauma center cared for the matriarch of a family that owned a giant corporation in a Central American country. This woman was accosted in the parking lot of a shopping mall and shot through the heart. She survived after a prolonged hospital course that included about a month in our surgical ICU. Her entire extended family and many friends came to our trauma center and held a vigil in our family area during her long stay. As our ICU contained twenty-five critically ill patients, we naturally had many other families present. So when the family of our VIP catered food for their friends and family, they generously provided wonderful cuisine for all the families at the trauma center. There was never a more positive atmosphere experienced at the trauma center than when fine food was supplied twenty-four hours a day for everybody. And after our VIP was discharged, her family donated a large sum of money for an endowed chair in trauma to help fund future pioneering investigative efforts.

Every day is a blessing.
STEPHEN M. COHN, M.D.

When I was an infant, my mother became deathly ill and went into acute renal failure (her kidneys stopped functioning). A previously healthy young woman, she probably had what we now call acute poststreptococcal glomerulonephritis. This is a form of renal failure that typically occurs in young children after strep infections and would today be treated by penicillin and maybe require short-term dialysis in some severe instances. But in the 1950s, dialysis was not available, and my mother was sent home to die with a serum creatinine of 9 (about ten times normal values). Think about it: she went home to say goodbye to my dad and her one-year-old son.

My father, then an intern at a residency program in Northern California, called up some of his old professors at the University of California, San Francisco medical school, and one recommended a new medication, prednisone. They gave my mother a shovelful of this steroid, blowing away her adrenal glands forever, but she survived. During those years, my grandmother, Rosie, helped take care of me. My mother never gained back all of her strength, but she never let her illness impact her desire to enjoy life and thrive. She was left with chronic venous stasis disease, as they had to use up all the veins, including those in her legs, to give her fluids and medications. She had paper-thin skin from the chronic steroids. If she bumped into anything, she sustained a huge wound on her leg that took months to heal.

When I was fresh out of fellowship in my first faculty position, I was very involved in animal physiology research and my clinical practice. One afternoon, my mom called me to chat. "How are things going with your science project?" she inquired. Feeling like a sixth grader who was completing his volcano demonstration for the science fair, I laughed loud and hard. "It's going great, Mom," I answered. So much for the "Big Docta." When she was in her late seventies, I got to hang with my mother for a week while my father had his aortic valve replaced. She was hilarious, so fun, and high energy. Each night when we would go out for dinner with friends, they would call me afterward, astonished at what a dynamic force and positive attitude she exuded. It was the first time I had spent time with her alone for decades. She lived to the age of eighty-five, always with a cheerful outlook. I can't remember her ever complaining about anything. Seriously. I guess when you are sent home to die, every day of life after that really is a blessing.

The blood is the life.

Book of Deuteronomy

A young construction worker was brought in to the trauma center after falling about 30 feet through a floor at a job site. He had a head injury, major chest wall injuries, and bilateral femur (thigh bone) fractures. We placed a breathing tube and chest tubes and notified the orthopedic service about his broken legs. Then it got interesting. The trauma social worker told me that there was a significant issue with the family. I was seated on a small sofa in the conference room reserved for family meetings. On one side of the room, the diminutive mother of the patient and the patient's new wife of two months were claiming that the injured party had recently become a Jehovah's Witness and should not receive transfused blood. On the other side of the room loomed the father and uncle. They stated in no uncertain terms that he was not a Jehovah's Witness and that we should give him all the blood he needed. In these matters, the wife's desires take priority as next of kin, so no blood transfusions would be given. A team of orthopedists came in immediately and fixed the patient's fractures. But over the next few days, the patient became progressively more anemic. A normal hemoglobin level is about 14 milligrams per deciliter (mg/dL), but the critical threshold is 5.5mg/dL, below which patients start to develop organ failure from not enough oxygen. His hemoglobin dropped to less than 4mg/dl, and he was dying. His organs were all failing. The father and uncle reached out to a friend, who was a judge, and obtained a temporary injunction. The critical care team transfused 10 units of blood overnight. The next day, the patient's wife got this judgment reversed, but by then he did not require any more blood. Most importantly, the patient survived.

Imagine that the circulation is a train containing the blood volume that is moving through the body, carrying oxygen to the tissues. If the red blood cells are train boxcars, the hemoglobin proteins can be thought of as small oxygen tanks contained in the train cars. During times of stress (such as exercise, injury, or infection), the tissues require more oxygen. The body can provide more oxygen by the heart pumping blood faster (enhanced heart rate increases the flow of blood) or by extracting more oxygen at the tissue level. Being anemic (having fewer train cars available to move oxygen) limits the oxygen accessible to the tissues. If the heart pump fails (the train slows down), or the blood oxygen content is decreased, like in severe COVID-19 pneumonia (fewer oxygen tanks), or the patient becomes severely anemic (not enough train cars), the body may lack adequate oxygen to sustain the tissues, and organ failure occurs.

Because trauma surgeons deal with a lot of bleeding, we are naturally quite interested in blood transfusion. About two-thirds of injured patients who survive to reach the hospital and then die do so from hemorrhage. And in the ICU, nearly all critically ill patients become anemic within a week.

The history of blood transfusion is truly fascinating. Most of physicians' work regarding blood through the ages has involved exsanguination (bloodletting) in a misguided effort to purify patients suffering from various illnesses. No one considered infusing blood until William Harvey first described circulation in the early 1600s. His contemporary, Christopher Wren, the legendary inventor and architect, experimented with ale, wine, and opium infusions into the bloodstreams of dogs via silver tubes. In 1667, Richard Lower in England and Jean-Baptiste Denys in France "successfully" infused blood from animals into humans. Unfortunately, these were primitive efforts with an unknown amount of blood infused via metal tubing from an immobilized animal (typically a calf or sheep) near the recipient. In an infamous case, a French nobleman died after repeated transfusions, and his wife sued Denys at the behest of the medical community for wrongful death. This court case received a huge amount of notoriety, as transfusionists were considered quacks in this era of bloodletting. The medical establishment was unified in its derision toward these practitioners. Denys was ultimately exonerated after it was shown that the patient's wife had poisoned him to death. However, medical societies across Europe established a moratorium against blood transfusion that lasted 150 years. Bloodletting was still the routine as evidenced as recently as 1799 when George Washington, one of the founding fathers of our country, died of a sore throat after his physicians removed over 2,300 cubic centimeters of blood (half of his blood volume) over about twelve hours. It was not until 1825, when English obstetrician James Blundell invented transfusion equipment, that blood transfusion experienced a rebirth, with human-to-human infusion. At the beginning of the twentieth century, researchers addressed many of the obstacles to blood transfusion, such as preventing blood from clotting with calcium salts and avoiding transfusion reactions with blood typing. Blood was infused by the semidirect transfusion method (where blood was removed into a receptacle, anticoagulated, and then infused later into a patient). These innovations along with rudimentary methods of blood preservation contributed to the formation of the first blood banks.

During World War I, blood transfusions were administered to a limited degree, particularly by Canadian military physicians. By the end of the war, the ability to provide 50 units of blood during a day was a sign of a quality field hospital. During World War II, blood became more readily available, but doctors did not consider it safe for storage for more than a few weeks, so little was infused until late in the war. Despite over 30,000 casualties per month, the Allies transfused fewer than 600,000 units of banked blood during the entire war. However, the lifesaving benefits of fresh whole blood were much appreciated by combat surgeons, and once these physicians returned to the United States, blood banks were created to meet their demands. Fast-forward to Operation Desert Storm in 1991, during which 82,000 units of blood were made available to the allied forces, but only about 250 units were required for the few casualties encountered.

The threshold for transfusion has changed over the last few decades as our knowledge of the physiological response to anemia has improved. While blood banks were desperate for blood in the late twentieth century, by 2014, the transfusion industry was shrinking. At that time, US demand for blood decreased by almost one-third in five years from 15 to 11 million units, despite an aging population. Almost all (95 percent) of the blood in storage in the United States is infused into about four million recipients. About two-thirds of the blood is used in the perioperative setting and one-third in emergency settings. Fewer than ten patients die each year from transfusion-related complications in North America, so blood is considered incredibly safe.

Analysis of blood use has revealed that most patients receive 1 to 2 units of blood and therefore could potentially have avoided receiving blood at all. These small-volume transfusions typically occur in patients who are bleeding in the operating room and the endpoint of hemorrhage is unpredictable. Some exsanguinating patients require more than 5 units, and this represents a large percentage of all the blood transfused. The amount of blood infused in any operation can be highly variable. (For example, one group reviewed one hundred thousand coronary bypass surgeries at four hundred centers and found that the infusion of blood varied depending on the specific medical center in 8 to 93 percent of their patients.[3])

There are many limitations to the use of blood. First, patients must undergo blood typing to avoid a transfusion reaction. While type O blood, the universal donor, can be given to anyone, type A and type B blood can only be given to individuals with the same blood type. The process of complete blood typing takes about forty-five minutes. In North America, about 40 percent of the population is type A and about 45 percent type O. Eleven percent of people are type B, and rarer types make up the remainder. Race and ethnicity impact blood type. Hispanic people are more likely to be type O. Asian people are predominantly type B.

Banked blood has a limited shelf life and outdates after forty-two days. So, to preserve the blood supply, when you arrive at the hospital bleeding to death, you will receive the oldest blood available in the blood bank. Blood deteriorates during storage, but older blood has not been demonstrated to be harmful clinically. Most important, blood is an immunosuppressive agent. In the 1960s, clinicians observed that more than 6 units of blood led to a significant improvement in kidney transplant graft survival. Prior transfusions made it less likely that the body would reject the kidney transplant.

In surgery and trauma, the development of infectious complications is related to the number of units of blood infused. Fortunately, infectious pathogens rarely contaminate the blood supply. This is because of the restricted blood donor pool and the myriad tests used to screen blood for HIV, hepatitis B and C, and other viral and bacterial organisms. By comparison, the risk of contracting hepatitis C (the most frequently occurring and dangerous of the pathogens) was 10 percent with 2 units of blood transfused in the late 1980s. Today the risk of hepatitis C with blood transfusion is less than one in a million. There is still the potential for a rare contaminant like Creutzfeldt-Jakob disease (mistakenly referred to as "mad cow" disease, which causes rapid death from neurological complications), Chagas disease (a rare parasitic infection affecting the heart), or more recently the Zika virus (which potentially impacts pregnancy).

One of the concerns regarding blood transfusion remains receiving the blood designated for another person and experiencing a transfusion reaction. This is a rare event and occurs in less than 1 in 14,000 units transfused. Recently, the risk of death from a blood transfusion was found to be about the same as death from a lightning strike (less than one per one million individuals) or about one-hundredth the likelihood of dying from a motor vehicle crash.[4]

Why do people become anemic? One reason is that healthcare providers are "medical vampires," meaning that we remove a lot of blood from our patients. Depending on where the patients are located and how easily we can access their bloodstream (indwelling catheters facilitate blood removal), we suck out a sizeable volume of blood from those under our care for various laboratory tests. This is particularly prevalent in the ICU, where blood sampling leads to anemia in most of our critically ill patients within a week of arrival. We used to transfuse our ICU patients whose hemoglobin level dropped to 10 (normal is about 14mg/dL). This was the standard of care for more than sixty years until investigators showed that a hemoglobin value of 7mg/dL was well tolerated even in those with a critical illness. Over the past twenty years, there have been a plethora of quality investigations among various populations (critically ill adults, critically ill children, cardiac surgery patients, hip surgery patients, patients with gastrointestinal bleeding, burn patients, and even patients with septic shock) that have all supported the notion that liberal transfusion strategies are not beneficial when compared to more restrictive management plans. This has led to a sharp reduction in blood use nationally. Hemoglobin values below 5.5mg/dL are associated with organ failure and are still to be avoided. This last bit of data was derived from the experience with a sizeable number of patients who refused blood transfusion (such as some Jehovah's Witnesses).

During critical illness, patients "like" to be anemic. By that, I mean that the body's normal physiological reaction is to permit or facilitate anemia. The primary stimulus to the production of new blood cells in the bone marrow in response to anemia is the production of erythropoietin (EPO). When we are very sick, not only do we not produce EPO in response to profound anemia; but if EPO is administered, we do not react to even pharmacologically high doses. So maybe there are some physiological or immunological advantages to being anemic when we are critically ill.

In trauma, a tiny proportion of our patients get a huge volume of blood. For example, according to a study from a major trauma center, 75 percent of all the blood transfused was given to just 3 percent of patients.[5] This "massive" transfusion used to be defined as 10 units of blood in twenty-four hours. Recently, this has been redefined as 3 or more units of blood required in an hour. This volume of blood seems to correlate with patient outcomes and signifies that the patient requires activation of a massive transfusion protocol (MTP). This process involves the blood bank and hospital resources converging to provide large volumes of blood and blood products (like plasma and platelets) for use by healthcare providers. During the infusion of large amounts of red blood cells to replace blood loss, we often need to provide other components of blood. Red cells in storage lack plasma (which contains most of our clotting factors) and platelets (a key blood component important in clotting blood). Therefore, during massive transfusion, we typically provide plasma and platelets in addition to the red cells.

If the clinician is unable to administer blood (due to patient choice) when needed, this can put the patient at considerable risk. For many years, I ran the bloodless (transfusion-free) center at my medical center. Our bloodless program functioned to ensure that patients who refused blood (such as many but not all Jehovah's Witnesses) received alternatives to transfusion. Members of the Jehovah's Witness religious community often refuse blood and blood products, but each church member has their own rules and desires. The healthcare team inquires of the patient, without family or clergy present, "Imagine we have a unit of blood in our hand. If you get it, you live; if you do not, you die. What do you want us to do?" Some of these patients say to give blood if it is essential, but not to tell anyone. I became interested in this subject because blood was often in short supply, so I conducted some research on blood substitutes in animal models and collaborated in some clinical trials. Fortunately, innovation by several creative clinician-scientists led to the development of transfusion avoidance and blood conservation methods. These principles have been applied to all our trauma and surgical patients, not just those refusing blood, and have helped reduce transfusions in the general population. A safe oxygen-carrying fluid alternative to blood is not yet available. Fortunately, the blood supply is much safer today than in decades past, as we have improved screening methods for a wide array of viral pathogens such as hepatitis and HIV.

Finally, the members of religious communities who refuse transfusions have forced us in the medical field to advance our understanding of the impact of anemia on human physiology. Many operations that historically were associated with significant blood loss and subsequent blood transfusion had to be modified for this population. In the process of learning how to minimize blood loss and find alternatives to the infusion of blood, the medical community, especially surgeons and anesthesiologists, had to be very innovative to ensure good patient outcomes. Most centers now have a bloodless medicine program that caters to the needs of patients refusing blood. There are a variety of techniques that are employed to avoid the development of severe anemia in the perioperative setting. In patients undergoing elective surgery, EPO is started well in advance of the operation. At the start of the operation, if permitted by the patient, 3 or 4 units are removed to a cell saver unit or into blood bags, which are maintained within a continuous circuit. Fluids are given to restore the loss of blood volume, and the case is conducted in a very anemic state. So any blood lost during surgery will have minimal red cells. In addition, during surgery, blood pressures are kept very low to decrease blood loss. At the end of the operation, the blood that was stored in the cell saver circuit or blood bags is then returned to the patient. Perioperatively, we avoid any blood draws. Using these and other techniques, surgical teams have completed operations historically associated with large amounts of blood loss, including liver transplantation and open-heart surgery. A few years ago, one of my research fellows focused his master's in public health thesis on trauma outcomes in a variety of religions with a particular interest in the Jehovah's Witness community. This group had significantly better outcomes than members of other religious groups who accept blood transfusion, possibly because of lifestyle and overall quality of health before injury.

A major difference between responsibility of
pilot and surgeon is that the former shares directly in
the consequences of his error or neglect,
while the latter does not.

JOHN S. LOCKWOOD (1907–1950)

In the middle of the night, I was operating on a young man who had been
shot in the abdomen. The operating scrub was a visiting nurse from Ire-
land. As we were completing our exploration and preparing to repair the

damage to the patient's duodenum (first part of the small bowel), she asked in her brogue, "Excuse me, doctor, is it customary for gang members to come to the operating theater?" Looking up, we saw a burly guy wearing a dark hoodie and a partially secured surgical mask charging into the OR. He was followed in a few seconds by a security guard. They began to wrestle along the operating room wall while the nurse pushed the OR table with all the surgical instruments back and forth to avoid contact. After a few minutes, they exited the room, still in a fighting embrace. Fortunately, no one was injured, and the patient survived without complications. In this unique and fortunately rare occurrence, the operating room we were using just happened to be situated directly across from a hospital elevator. This visitor, who had somehow eluded security, turned out to be from the same gang as the patient and was just checking on the status of his buddy.

Rarely do surgeons place themselves intentionally in harm's way. Even in the military, it makes little sense to put a limited resource on the front line where a mortar round can take out the lone surgeon supporting many soldiers. However, sometimes we come close. Hospital security must separate some of our trauma patients from their weapons to keep the environment safe, particularly at inner-city urban trauma centers. On one occasion, a patient who had been injured in a munitions factory explosion was transported by helicopter to the trauma center. He was brought immediately to the operating room. After clearing the space of any personnel, one of my partners removed a live rocket-propelled grenade (RPG) embedded in his abdomen. This is a freak occurrence, particularly in the civilian world, but amazingly, two of my former fellows had removed these RPGs from patients in the war zones of Afghanistan and

Iraq. (I am told these are extremely rare cases in modern military history.) And I once met a Red Cross surgeon who claimed to have removed a live grenade from the thorax of a patient in Cambodia in the 1960s (this experience was portrayed in the movie *The Killing Fields*).

During training, one of my fellow residents, Frank Pomposelli, related to me a story he had heard about one of his compadres. Two gang members were brought into the ER from a major altercation and placed on adjoining stretchers in the trauma resuscitation area. One man died despite all attempts to save him. Upon seeing his friend die, the other individual leaped from his stretcher, whipped out a switchblade, and cornered the emergency room nurses and surgeons. A passing medical student saw this happening and, thinking quickly, charged a defibrillator and shocked the assailant into submission. We would say that this student was definitely "surgical material." I am told that he went on to complete a surgical residency.

> *It is a good thing for a physician to have prematurely gray hair and itching piles (hemorrhoids). The first makes him appear to know more than he does, and the second gives him an expression of concern, which the patient interprets as being on his behalf.*
>
> A. BENSON CANNON (1889–1950)

I was giving a talk to second-year medical students with the trauma program manager, who was a senior nurse. I started by telling them that trauma cases and emergency care were nothing like what they were watching on a popular TV series at that time, ER. *The students were shocked when I added, "But the dysfunctional interpersonal relationships were very accurate." The nurse confirmed.*

You never want to watch a medical TV show or movie with me. I am the guy constantly railing about inaccuracies. My kids used to complain that I was ruining the shows, so I just stopped watching. One of my biggest TV or movie pet peeves is when surgeons are shown digging around in wounds to retrieve bullets. Surgeon John Hunter condemned this activity in the late 1700s, and it is not something we do. If we run across a bullet in our operative exploration, we will give it to the police as evidence. Occasionally, if a bullet becomes irritating or leads to an infection (a rare occurrence), we can excise them. If it is floating in the heart or occluding a blood vessel, it needs to be removed in a formal operation. Otherwise, 99 percent of the time, we leave bullets alone. They typically don't do anything. And nobody ever blindly jams a clamp down a hole and goes fishing for a projectile.

The other irritating thing is that everyone on TV dies instantly. Either they bleed out, or they suffocate in about five seconds. Nobody dies that fast unless you are decapitated or your heart is ripped in half. I was watching the movie *The Transporter*, and there is a scene where a villain pushes a handkerchief into the back of a person's throat, and they expire in no time (they struggled for a few seconds and then . . . gone). This process takes minutes, not seconds.

And what is a "medically induced coma" that every TV patient seems to undergo? This procedure would be an exceedingly rare event, where we sedate and paralyze a patient with medications to induce a coma. But it seems like everyone in the TV hospitals has this procedure, maybe because it sounds so awful.

In the 1980s, we put patients on special ICU beds that tilted slowly from side to side—the RotoRest bed—to improve lung function, help clear secretions, and avoid pressure ulcers. (Imagine lying in a kayak as it sways from side to side and back and forth.) Late one night, we transported a very intoxicated trauma patient into an ICU filled with patients rocking back and forth slowly on these beds. The unit was dark except for the monitors flashing. At the time, the most popular movie in theaters was *Coma*. In his inebriated state, our patient started to freak out, thinking he was in the film, about to be put into a "medically induced coma" and have his organs harvested.

If TV programs showed people how our work is performed, they would not be dramatic enough. The fact is the best clinicians always keep their cool. The worse things get, the calmer you must become as a trauma surgeon—and not faking your serenity but being like an ice cube. Wouldn't you want your pilot to remain calm in a catastrophe, the way Captain Sully Sullenberger was landing on the Hudson? In the emergency center or the operating room, the entire trauma team takes cues from the trauma team leader. And some of these situations are hairy, but we must remain tranquil. One of my colleagues in Chicago told me about appearing on a reality TV trauma surgery series filmed in his trauma center. Each week, his mother would call and criticize his performance, as he always remained calm and credible, often predicting poor patient outcomes, while the chief resident was upbeat and optimistic. His mother's friends felt he was not a good surgeon because he was not excessively cheerful and energized. But that is reality.

Because of the uncontrolled nature of trauma and the uncertainty of what we will encounter, a calm work environment is essential. It is not surprising that a hysterical or frantic trauma team is not conducive to the smooth and effective management of patients with unknown and unpredictable injuries. While I was in residency, an unresponsive patient with a severe head injury was undergoing resuscitation when his entire blood volume squirted out of his left ear onto the wall. His heart stopped immediately, and he died. Such a rapid demise after surviving to reach the hospital is relatively rare. In another instance, a car driver was brought by a helicopter from a car crash. He had blood all over him and an extremely low blood pressure. As we gave him blood and fluids and his blood pressure improved, he started to bleed profusely from his neck and head. We learned later that the patient had been driving at highway speeds when he was stabbed multiple times by a man in the back seat before crashing the vehicle. (Turns out the assailant's wife was riding in the front passenger seat, and he suspected she was having an affair with the driver.) As the patient began to expel blood like a shower nozzle from his head and neck, we discovered that he had been stabbed and that the shaft of the knife had been broken off in his neck and was embedded in his spine. He only survived for about twenty-four hours. Unfortunately, making a television show enjoyable requires the writers to accelerate the treatment processes' speed and accentuate the caretakers' emotional lability.

Back in the days of carrying the "code beeper," there was an overhead page for "Dr. Standstill to the Bank." "Dr. Standstill" was hospital speak for a "code blue," or a cardiac arrest, but where was the Bank? I had to find my way across a long overhead bridge covering a four-lane avenue to reach the commercial bank that adjoined the hospital proper. I arrived at

about the same time as a cardiology fellow and an anesthesia fellow push-
ing a code cart (a large mobile box containing all the resuscitation equip-
ment). A young man was lying in front of the bank entrance, not
breathing and without a pulse. Our team worked like a well-oiled
machine: the anesthesiologist put in a breathing tube, I inserted a central
venous catheter (to gain access to his bloodstream for medications), and
someone pumped on his chest. We put on the ECG leads and saw he was
in ventricular fibrillation, a serious and often terminal cardiac rhythm.
We charged up the defibrillator. "Everybody clear," said the cardiology
fellow, who fired the paddles. There was a jerk as the electrical current
went through the patient, then suddenly, "We have a pulse" and "He is
back in sinus" (meaning he now had normal heart electrical activity).
There was a loud murmur around us. We looked up to see a massive
crowd of bank onlookers peering over our shoulders at real medicine in
action. We all wanted to say, "It never happens like this." Because it
never does. We run hundreds of codes without a survivor (the survival
rate for out-of-hospital cardiac arrest is only about 4 percent). But this
was just like on TV . . .

> *Surgeons and anatomists see no beautiful*
> *women in their lives, but only a ghastly stack*
> *of bones with Latin names to them.*
>
> MARK TWAIN (1835–1910)

Young, single, and fresh out of training, I was walking through the
radiology department one day when a beautiful woman working in front
of a wall of X-rays looked up and gave me a radiant smile. "Hello, Dr. C,"
she said. "Hello," I answered, flustered that I had no idea who she was.
"You don't recognize me? I am Karen B," she said. "That is not possible,"

I replied. Karen B was a young patient I had treated a few years previously after a car crash resulting in a significant head injury and multiple fractures. She was now unrecognizable, with a full head of hair (it had been shaved off for her brain surgery), makeup, and no breathing tube or skeletal traction.

I have heard that some folks leave the house in their best undergarments to guarantee that they look their best should they end up in the emergency room. We do not ever notice what anyone looks like when we cut off their clothes in a trauma case. I once was out at brunch with a fellow and his wife when he exclaimed, "I heard you saved Miss (US state) the other day." He had taken care of her in the ICU after surgery. I said that I had taken care of no such person. He was, in fact, correct. A woman had arrived, having almost been cut in half when her limo struck a tractor-trailer. It was the end of the day, and as I walked out to my car through the trauma area, they were rolling her through the entry doors covered in blood. I dropped everything and joined the trauma surgeon on call to resuscitate the patient. She was gravely ill and barely survived a massive laceration through her chest (imagine being struck with a broadsword like in the movie *Braveheart*) with her shoulder almost cut off. Her aorta (the major blood vessel from the heart to the body) was torn, and she experienced multiple cardiac arrests during surgery. After a series of operations, she survived, but none of us knew of her lovely appearance. I have heard that she is now a motivational speaker.

I should clarify that the trauma team and the trauma surgeon rarely have any idea about the outcomes of patients after they recover and initiate their rehabilitation process. Most of these patients are seen by orthopedists following their fracture or ligament repairs or by neurosurgeons after spine or brain surgery. The doctors at the rehabilitation facilities and the physical therapists are the primary caretakers during the recuperation process. Finally, patients are referred to their primary care physicians when they return home. General/trauma surgeons only have a brief follow-up if there are issues regarding the coordination of care or complications. We rarely have any knowledge of our patients' long-term consequences of injury.

> *Every idea is an incitement . . . eloquence*
> *may set fire to reason.*
>
> OLIVER WENDELL HOLMES JR. (1841–1935)

My daughter Elizabeth, the standup comedian, does a bit where she describes riding on an airplane with me while an entire girls' soccer team around me was getting grossed out by the photos on my laptop. In her version, I am reviewing gory slides of injured genitalia (which never happened). But I often have some graphic trauma photos that I rifle through as part of my preparation for lectures I give.

On more than one occasion, I have been asked to perform some medical care while on a passenger jet. In one instance, an older man sitting next to me dropped his book as the flight reached cruising altitude. I realized that he was unconscious and spent the entire flight giving him critical care, assessing his vital signs, administering oxygen, and inserting an IV for some fluids. I knelt next to him for about sixty minutes. After landing in Atlanta, the paramedics came aboard and took him to the hospital. I never heard another word from the airline or the patient.

But sometimes, good things come out of being a Good Samaritan. On a flight to Ft. Lauderdale, we stopped in Washington, DC, to pick up passengers. While they were loading, a man had a generalized seizure. I walked to the aisle where he was convulsing. Another passenger standing over him asked, "Are you a physician?" When I said yes, he asked, "What type?" I thought that was a strange question, but I said I was a surgeon and intensivist. "Great," he said, relieved. "I am a psychiatrist, and I have not treated a seizure in over ten years." This psychiatrist, Dave, and I managed to care for the patient until the EMTs arrived. On landing in Florida, my family rented a car and drove to a resort where, who did we meet? Dave and his family. We became fast friends after spending the entire week vacationing together. He even taught me how to water ski (but left me in the swamp with the alligators for a scary couple of minutes). Dave continues to tell everyone, jokingly, that he bailed me out managing the patient on the plane. . . . He is clearly delusional.

Surgeons are sometimes asked to work on a temporary or vacation coverage basis. This is referred to as locum tenens, per diem, or moonlighting. During my fellowship, I performed this type of work to make some extra income, but I rarely did this as a surgical faculty member. One summer, shortly after I finished my fellowship training, I was asked to provide weekend coverage for the vacationing general surgeon at a hospital on Martha's Vineyard. They would include an auto pass for the ferry (impossible to get), a stipend, and accommodations. All I had to do was carry the beeper, and I could go anywhere on the island as long as I could return to the hospital easily if needed. Sounded like a vacation with pay . . .

I arrived at Martha's Vineyard on a gorgeous summer day and was given a quick orientation at the small hospital. They showed me around and then handed me a beeper that went off as it was placed in my hand. The digital number was for the hospital emergency room. I went down to find an older man in septic shock with peritonitis and an abdominal abscess affecting his kidney. He needed an emergency operation, which I performed before moving the patient to the tiny ICU. I managed his critical illness from the bedside for the next seventy-two hours, using all of the most advanced monitoring catheters and medications. I did not leave his bedside other than to grab food or use the bathroom and had little sleep the entire weekend. On Monday morning, he had stabilized but was still very sick on the ventilator. I packed up to leave and started to say farewell when the nurse administrator said, "Where are you going and what are we supposed to do with him?" There was no one coming in to care for such a patient. So I arranged for him to be flown to my university hospital for me to care for after I drove to the ferry and then home from my excellent "holiday" on Martha's Vineyard.

Det som inte dödar, härdar [What doesn't kill, hardens].

SWEDISH PROVERB

We were on a college graduation trip in the northern part of Sweden, trying our hand at mushing. A disaster was in the making as a driverless dog sled with my daughter Claudia zipped up inside the cargo basket plummeted downhill. The sled became momentarily airborne as the animals whipped around the corner and out of sight. At the start of this adventure, our guide/instructor imparted a single rule for the drivers,

"Do not let go of the sled." But the teams of Alaskan huskies were revved up and ready to start, and unfortunately, we were on a slab of ice at the top of a hill. As the dogs lunged forward, Claudia's boyfriend lost control and fell off the sled as it shot forward. My wife and I were waiting by the next sled and were worried that Claudia would sustain a brain injury (or worse). Fortunately, no contact occurred between the sled and the surrounding trees as it flew down the hillside. Claudia had made it down the hill unscathed. After that, she drove the sled . . .

Then it was our turn, with my wife excited to mush the wild beasts (the dogs, not me). But I outweighed my wife by 100 pounds, and we were on a frozen hill. So when she stood on the brakes, nothing happened, and the sled shot forward and flipped on a boulder. The metal whacked her foot hard, breaking multiple bones. She toughed it out for a couple of hours in the sled, but the pain in her foot worsened. It was time to experience the Swedish healthcare system, which was impressive. After driving over two hours to the nearest hospital, we were quickly seen by their busy but courteous staff. We were informed before my wife was even evaluated that our bill would be 414 US dollars as visitors to Sweden. Four hundred and fourteen dollars? This included multiple evaluations by the emergency room doctor: X-rays and spiral CT scans of the foot, the work of a cast team to immobilize the injury (three broken bones in her foot), and a pair of high-tech crutches. The crutches alone would have cost that amount in the United States.

From an injury perspective, it is interesting to note the differences in the perception of risk and personal responsibility that we have observed in other countries. While in Iceland for a short winter visit, we noticed tourists in wetsuits submerging into frozen lakes. As an experienced diver, I asked our guide if this was risky in extremely frigid conditions. He said matter-of-factly that yes, a couple of visitors had died the previous week during their frozen underwater adventure. Subsequently, we visited a huge, beautiful waterfall with an ice-covered path across the outlook. We cringed as we watched slow-moving older folks trudging across supported only by their canes. There was no railing, so one slip and over she goes! So injury risk and responsibility for injury prevention are handled much differently in different parts of the globe.

> *Persons who are naturally very fat are apt*
> *to die earlier than those who are slender.*
>
> HIPPOCRATES (460–377 BCE)

Americans continue to get bigger and bigger, making our jobs as surgeons that much more difficult. One of my chief residents told the story of operating on an exceptionally large woman who needed her gallbladder removed. Before the era of laparoscopy, this was often done through a horizontal incision under the right rib cage. During this procedure, because of the patient's massive girth, the surgeons missed the abdomen and struck the operative table.

Surgeons hate to operate on patients with a large amount of body fat. The exception, of course, are the bariatric surgeons. They, by definition, work on this part of the population to shrink them down to the size where we can manage their various medical problems. Unfortunately, the public keeps getting larger. According to the CDC, from 1999–2000 through 2017–2018, US obesity prevalence increased from 30.5 percent to 42.4 percent. During the same time, the prevalence of severe obesity increased from 4.7 percent to 9.2 percent. This means that almost half of our patients are obese now, and one in four is estimated to be severely obese by 2030.[6]

It is much, much harder to operate on someone who is even 50 pounds overweight. First, exposure of the operative site is very problematic in open surgical cases. The tissues are often more friable and prone to bleeding. Fat can engulf organs, making them harder to dissect. And even laparoscopy is more complicated, as it is much harder to gain safe entry into the abdominal cavity due to the thickness of the fat-filled abdominal wall. At one hospital where I worked, the trauma service was called to the OR to manage a morbidly obese patient who had slid off the operating table and struck their head. And even bariatric surgeons can have issues. About twenty-five years ago, one of my partners performed a bariatric operation on a man weighing well over 500 pounds. The surgeon's rule was that all her patients were expected to walk the night after the operation. The problem was that when the patient was returning to bed, he missed the edge and slid down to sit on the hospital floor. The healthcare team had to call 911 so a fire rescue squad could come and hoist him back onto the bed, as his weight exceeded the hospital's bedside lifting equipment limits.

And once the operations on the obese are completed, it is much more difficult to safely close the abdomen, which is prone to breaking open after surgery (called fascial dehiscence). Fat does not have a good blood supply, so wound infections significantly increase in this population. Then there are all the postoperative respiratory complications. Patients who are overweight are harder to mobilize after surgery and are therefore more likely to have venous clots form in their extremities. Long term, the likelihood of an incisional hernia (a weakness or bulge at the incision site that can contain abdominal contents) requiring surgical intervention is higher in the heavy patient.

In addition to performing trauma and emergency surgery, many trauma surgeons have an elective practice where we operate on patients in a planned or elective fashion. Prior to elective surgery on obese patients, I place them on exercise programs with diets to help them lose weight and improve surgical outcomes. Remarkably, with a simple walking program (reaching about 2 miles per day) and some help from nutritionists regarding food choices, patients were able to lose about 1 pound a week for a year or two. Some folks lost almost 100 pounds before surgery. Unfortunately, many of these obese patients are introduced to us when they need an emergency procedure, so there is no time for a weight loss program. Thus, it should be clear that obesity is harmful beyond merely affecting people's health in terms of cardiovascular and joint stress. In addition, considerable danger may be incurred when undergoing many types of surgery.

> *A question that sometimes drives me hazy:*
> *am I or are the others crazy?*
> ALBERT EINSTEIN (1879–1955)

"Blood has been dripping on my head all night," said the patient. We were at a busy city hospital, and many of our patients were withdrawing from drug or alcohol addiction or were mentally ill. I was concerned that this patient was hallucinating. His statement led to a head bob from me as the chief resident to a junior resident, which signified we needed to consult psychiatry stat. However, when we visited the ICU on the floor above, we found that a patient with cirrhosis of the liver had been

bleeding from his GI tract all night and that there was a massive puddle
of blood under his bed. Blood was seeping through the floor, causing
drops of blood to land on the patient on the floor below.

I could fill this book with stories about things that people do that
we would all judge to be mentally unbalanced. Like the young guy
during my residency years who decided to reside under a bridge
during the coldest days of the year in Boston (despite pockets full
of money). He arrived at the ER frozen (hypothermic with severe
frostbite) and later that week required amputation of all four
extremities because of an overwhelming infection. Integrating
trauma care with the psychiatry service is undoubtedly a challenge, as doing something bizarre does not necessarily constitute a
danger to yourself or others or require involuntary psychiatric
commitment. But when someone is deemed appropriate to undergo
psychiatric care in a specialized facility, their medical issues must
be resolved and their injuries healed before being referred to a psychiatric facility. So you can imagine that many unusual people
(including the doctors) populate the trauma service.

The psychiatric patient had been seen in the ER a few days previously
with an infected foot. He had either elected to leave AMA (against med-
ical advice) or had just run off. On this day, he was barely responsive,
with his diabetes out of control and pus now draining from his gangre-
nous foot. He was so unstable that the decision was made to place a
breathing tube and move him to the ICU, where I was the junior resi-
dent, to correct his metabolic state before taking him to the operating
room. After he arrived at the ICU, his vital signs deteriorated, and we
realized that because his foot had wet gangrene, we had to perform

surgery at the bedside to save his life. Imagine this picture. . . . It is night-time, and we are on the top floor of the city hospital, which has wall-sized glass windows and skylights. We were experiencing a monster storm with thunder reverberating and multiple lightning flashes. As we started to saw off the patient's leg, there was a giant thunderclap, and all the electricity went out. We completed amputating his leg in pitch black under the beam of a flashlight with occasional lightning flashes. Shades of Frankenstein! In the morning, his physiology restored, the patient jumped out of bed and tried to escape the unit on his stump.

> *A ship under sail and a big-bellied woman are the handsomest two things that can be seen common.*
>
> BENJAMIN FRANKLIN (1706–1790)

Sometimes, the life of a mother is preserved to sustain the life of a fetus. When I was a resident, we treated a young pregnant woman with HIV who had a massive stroke and was declared brain dead. She was early in her second trimester, so her fetus was not capable of surviving if delivered at that stage of development. For many months, we maintained the physiological functions of this woman who was officially dead so that her baby could be delivered safe and sound. This occurred via cesarean section after her long ICU course.

Probably the most hazardous type of trauma we see is an injury occurring during pregnancy. We must sustain the life of the pregnant woman as well as her baby. Motor vehicle–related injuries remain the leading cause of death among women of reproductive age. Motor vehicle crashes during pregnancy are the leading cause of traumatic fetal mortality and serious maternal injury morbidity and mortality in the United States, injuring more than two hundred thousand pregnant women each year, with three thousand to five thousand fetal deaths.

Seat belt use reduces the risk of adverse maternal and fetal outcomes throughout pregnancy. The current recommendation is very specific as to wearing the shoulder belt between the breasts and wearing the lap belt low across the upper thighs, as this positioning distributes the force of the impact and reduces the risk of injury to both the mother and fetus. Not unexpectedly, pregnancy makes women more susceptible to abdominal injury from car collisions.

On one occasion, a woman who was very advanced in her pregnancy was locked out of her apartment late at night. She attempted to enter via the third-floor balcony of her neighbor. This required her to jump from one railing to another, which was quite difficult considering her huge girth. She fell two stories and arrived to the ER in shock from blood loss. We immediately assessed the mother and baby and found the baby to be in severe distress. This was not about choosing mother or baby; they were both about to die. As we intubated the mother and initiated her resuscitation, we performed an emergency cesarean section right there in the trauma resuscitation area and then handed the nearly lifeless baby off to the neonatal ICU doctors. The mother was moved immediately to the operating room to deal with her major injuries. While the mother survived, sadly, the baby did not, despite all of our efforts. Fortunately, this type of tragedy is a rare event.

One of the most dreaded types of injuries that occurs most typically in the second and third trimesters is placental abruption, which is when the placenta essentially peels off the uterine lining, preventing blood flow to the fetus. Think of Velcro slowly being peeled off a surface. If the fetus is not carefully monitored for signs of placental abruption (slowing of heart rate), the lack of oxygen can result in the death of the fetus.

Sometimes, even after delivery, the wheels can fall off. One woman developed a bad infection in her uterus (endometritis) following an emergency cesarean section and required an emergency hysterectomy. She was taken to the operating room in septic shock. The procedure was particularly difficult, as she had developed liver dysfunction and was not clotting normally. Added to that, her obstetrician-gynecologist injured one of the large iliac veins in her pelvis during the hysterectomy, leading to massive bleeding. That was when we, the trauma surgeons, were called to stem the hemorrhage. Unfortunately, the stress of sepsis and massive bleeding led to the rupturing of a leaflet of the patient's mitral valve, which required the placement of an intra-aortic balloon pump to support her heart function. Therefore, this patient had septic, hemorrhagic, and cardiogenic shock all at the same time. After a difficult ICU course, she survived.

When I was an intrepid medical student, we were tasked to deliver babies at what was then the busiest delivery hospital in the United States (more than sixteen thousand babies delivered a year). This hospital no longer exists. This was my first clinical rotation, and I was one of the handful of students who were assigned to be on call the very first night of the eight-week rotation. The job of the medical student was to place intravenous catheters and monitor the women in labor while we waited for our chance to "catch" a newborn. Uncomplicated pregnancies were all handled by a medical student and a nurse alone. We responded in rotation to shouts of "DELIVERY" by the fortunately highly experienced nurses, and we ran to one of the labor rooms. "Hurry up and scrub, the baby is coming," I was told by the nurse for my first delivery. That morning, we had spent some time in an operating room learning how to scrub. The standard in those days was ten minutes of scrubbing with ten strokes on each surface of each finger and palm and lower arm. I was counting down as I scrubbed each surface, "5, 4, 3, 2 . . ." for a few minutes when the nurse popped her head in the door and stated, "We need you for this delivery." I responded, "9, 8, 7, 6, I am almost done." A few seconds later, she yelled, "Right now, or this baby will deliver itself." I ran into the room, slapped on a gown, and managed to struggle into one glove when out popped the baby. I barehanded the baby, cut the cord, and handed off the healthy little person to the labor and delivery nurse. She looked hard at me over her mask and scolded me. "Doctor, these babies are not going to wait for you." I learned my lesson. A year later, I was asked to work during a holiday when some of the senior students were allowed to fill in to earn a few dollars. That day, I delivered twenty-four healthy babies in twenty-four hours.

One of my trauma surgeon colleagues was traveling to the hospital with his wife, who was in advanced labor with their third child. Traffic was so heavy in Manhattan that afternoon that the taxi was making no progress. Fortunate to have a physician husband and an experienced cab driver, she delivered a lovely baby boy, Sheldon, right there in the back seat. Apparently, this is so common in New York City that there is a checkbox listed on the birth certificate for "taxicab" as the location of birth.

8

PREVENTING INJURIES

Today surgeons and psychiatrists use drugs more
than ever before. In their overuse and misuse lie many
of the misfires of all medical care.
FRANCIS D. MOORE (1913–2001)

In the late 1990s, I fell while inline skating and broke my leg. After sur-
gery, I received patient-controlled analgesia with a narcotic, which made
me nauseous. I was then given a new long-acting opioid drug, OxyCon-
tin, at the lowest possible dose twice a day. After five days, I became
convinced that I was not getting pain relief, so I decided to stop taking the
drug and skipped my 6 p.m. dose. The next morning, I crutched out to
my partner's car for a ride to work in the morning. During the entire
thirty-minute ride, all I could think was "I will feel better if I take one of
those little white pills." And then, for the entire hour of morning report,
when all the cases from the day before were presented, I could not listen
to anything, as all I could think was "I will feel better if I take one of
those little white pills." I went to my office and could not concentrate on
reading my emails. I realized I was going through opioid withdrawal

and tossed the pills. I crutched around the medical center until 1 p.m.
that afternoon, more than thirty hours after the last dose, before I could
concentrate on anything but taking another of "those little white pills."
No wonder patients arrive at the office taking monster doses of this stuff
every day. OxyContin (and opioids in general) is incredibly addictive.

Death from opioid overdose is now considered a national emergency. According to the CDC, more than five hundred thousand Americans have perished because of narcotic overdose since 1999. Physicians prescribing opioids, particularly in the perioperative period, are significant contributors to narcotic addiction. Nonopioid medications such as ibuprofen (brand name Motrin) are equivalent to narcotics (such as oxycodone) in controlling both acute pain[1] and chronic pain[2] without becoming addictive. In Europe, narcotics are not typically prescribed after surgery. This practice remains commonplace, however, in the United States. My colleagues and I recently reviewed the side effects of ibuprofen and the family of drugs called NSAIDs (nonsteroidal anti-inflammatory drugs) and found that the risks often advertised to the prescribers are negligible when used for a brief period, even in high-risk patients.[3] In trauma, we try to avoid narcotics and aim to discharge our patients on alternatives to these dangerous, addictive opioid drugs.

"One hundred and sixty-four," he said as he woke up after a shot of Narcan (the opioid reversal agent). That was the exact number of opioid containers (plastic packets about the size of a 12-gauge shotgun slug, 2.5 inches long by .75 inches across) that this South American drug mule had ingested before getting on a plane to Miami. Failure to produce the exact number of capsules would result in death for the drug runner and their

family. The transporter had arrived at the trauma center in a coma because a heroin-filled capsule had exploded in his intestines and was absorbed into his bloodstream. We brought the patient to the operating room to remove all the packets in his GI tract that we could find. An escort of Drug Enforcement Administration agents perched like vultures in the room, watching our every move. Fortunately, we retrieved most of the drug pods, and the rest passed the natural way.

> *Those diseases which medicines do not cure, iron cures; those which iron cannot cure, fire cures; and those which fire cannot cure, are to be reckoned wholly incurable.*
>
> HIPPOCRATES (460–377 BCE)

In the previous section, I related my experience with nearly immediate dependence on OxyContin, which I recognized after about five days and stopped right away. My episode of near addiction to opioids and similar experiences of many other people resulted in part from misinformation spread by drug representatives from the pharmaceutical industry claiming that this particular "nonaddicting narcotic" characterized a special class of drugs approved by the Food and Drug Administration (FDA). As shown on the TV miniseries *Dopesick*, the claim that OxyContin was "addicting to less than 1 percent of recipients" by the pharmaceutical companies was false. The fact that doctors accepted that a narcotic was nonaddicting as the truth, just because the FDA or a drug representative claimed this, defied common sense. But it is difficult for busy practicing clinicians to take the time to dig deeply into clinical trials to look for safety and efficacy (proof that the product works), particularly when experts in the field are supporting these claims.

The pharmaceutical companies realized years ago that they could market their wares to surgeons in the late twentieth century using attractive salespeople. You could pick the drug reps out of a group, as they were the best-dressed, most engaging lovely ladies and handsome men encountered in an office or medical center setting. In 1987, an affair with a pharmaceutical drug rep, Donna Rice, derailed the presidential campaign of former senator Gary Hart. Ms. Rice had won the Miss South Carolina World beauty pageant and was an actress on the TV series *Miami Vice*. Exactly the kind of woman that could open doors of doctors' offices or party with politicians. Many of these drug reps would offer physicians fine dinners, and they often had a handful of tickets to major sports or theater events. Busy surgeons were flattered by the attention of these gorgeous creatures and were happy to try new products. Realizing that the drug manufacturers were doing all they could to try to bias us to use their products, I made it my practice decades ago to demand the data behind any claim before prescribing any drug or device to my patients or those on my service. I have tried to maintain vigilance in this area.

An example of adoption of a nonsense product encouraged by pharmaceutical reps is the use of "biologic meshes." When patients develop an incisional hernia (a defect in the strong fascial layer of the abdominal wall that often occurs after an abdominal operation), these bulges can enlarge and become symptomatic. Sometimes a loop of bowel can become stuck in this space and require emergency surgery. Based on zero data, biologic meshes—made of an organic product like a sheep's intestine—were touted as being safer and more effective than a piece of plastic mesh, which was our standard for repairing these hernias in the elective setting.

The biologic meshes are hugely expensive (sometimes more than $50,000 for a single operation) compared with the few hundred dollars for most synthetic mesh products. How did these biologic meshes get approved by the FDA? The manufacturers of devices (mesh is considered a device, not a drug) are only required to show that they resemble another product existing on the market. So once a single biologic mesh had been approved decades ago, others could join the melee. Soon, there were many of these biologic mesh products available. In my experience and that of my colleagues, these meshes did not work, and they led to more infections in the wound and dissolved, leaving the hernia defect unchanged. So we stopped using them. But for more than thirty years, they were claimed to be as valuable as and superior to plastic mesh. Why didn't we conduct a clinical trial to study this issue? The answer is, we tried. If an investigator wants to do a randomized trial comparing two products (say, biologic mesh with plastic mesh for abdominal wall hernias), they must provide both meshes free to the patient. They also must get FDA approval from the company to use its product in a clinical trial, something called an IDE (investigational device exemption). The astronomical cost of the biologic mesh made this process too expensive for most researchers to finance outside of a large federal grant. And, of course, the manufacturers did not want a study to be performed, as it might show that their cash cow was not effective. In the last couple of years, for the first time, randomized trials (studies that alternate who gets one product or the other by random chance) have proven clearly that biologic meshes are not as effective as plastic meshes. Biologic meshes are hopefully not being used much today.

One of the best examples of this aggressive corporate marketing approach was the advertising campaign of Factor 7a. In 1999, a case published in a prestigious medical journal discussed the use of a blood component, Factor 7a, to stop bleeding in an Israeli soldier.[4] This patient had been injured in combat and had been infused with many units of blood and blood products. In a last-ditch effort to salvage his life, a hematologist administered a medication used primarily for hemophilia (a genetic bleeding disorder in which the blood doesn't clot properly—these patients lack specific proteins to clot, i.e., Factor 8 or Factor 9). When hemophiliacs receive enough of these factors over time, they become resistant, and Factor 7a can be used to help the patient's blood clot. But using Factor 7a in a trauma patient was utterly novel. This soldier had likely developed a bleeding disorder because the clinicians had diluted many of his clotting factors.

The manufacturer of Factor 7a, a Scandinavian company known for producing insulin for diabetics, developed an aggressive marketing campaign to use its product in bleeding trauma patients. The drug was hugely expensive (nearly $20,000 a dose) and was just a few years from coming off-patent (generic drugs are often much cheaper). So full-page advertisements for Factor 7a began appearing in our major trauma journal as it related to its use in hemophilia. We thought this odd, as it is estimated that fewer than thirty-three thousand people in the United States have this rare genetic disorder. But clinicians began clamoring to give Factor 7a to bleeding trauma patients. Hospital administrators became quite concerned, as there are a very large number of trauma patients, so this represented a potentially huge expenditure. To the manufacturer's credit, some clinical trials were funded. The safety profile of Factor 7a was not found to be particularly favorable, and there appeared to be some increase in thrombotic complications (such as stroke or heart attack) in some studies. And only very rarely do trauma patients develop a refractory coagulopathy (medical bleeding). The drug is very rarely used in trauma today.

> *When all those around you are losing their heads,*
> *you are perfectly calm. . . . You probably don't*
> *understand the magnitude of the situation!*
>
> My father, Leland Henry Cohn, M.D.,
> reversing the saying of Rudyard Kipling

In May 2020, I got a phone call from a former surgical colleague living in Arizona. She and her ER doctor husband wanted to know if all this pandemic stuff was a left-wing media fantasy. I said, "Dude, during this short phone call, I was texted that two of my ICU patients with COVID had died." It was no joke.

In the spring of 2020, the coronavirus disease swept through New York City and the surrounding area and wreaked havoc on the populace. No wonder. We knew people in our apartment building who had flown from Paris with a planeload of folks from Asia and Italy to JFK Airport in early March, with zero screening on arrival. They had all simply dispersed into the general New York population. I have a photo of Madison Avenue at midday later that month, without a car or human in sight.

Trauma surgeons are all trained as ICU physicians, but they typically limit their care to the surgical ICU. Suddenly, we had over five hundred critically ill COVID patients in our hospital on a given day, so many of us surgeons became medical ICU doctors. This was particularly difficult because no one understood how to treat the disease, and protective gear was limited. At that time, the data from Europe was that the death rate was over 90 percent for COVID patients requiring a ventilator. Three of my ten trauma surgeon partners contracted significant cases of the virus, and one ended up in one of our own ICUs.

We would deliver patient care for hours in poorly laid-out makeshift ICUs (even turning our cafeteria and offices into space for medical beds), and regular patient rooms were repurposed as ICUs. And as we walked around the hospital floor, patients would die. During a week of coverage, it was not unusual for twenty patients to expire, two to be discharged out of the ICU, and the rest to remain gravely ill. To give context, it was rare for patients to die in the surgical ICU before COVID-19 unless care had been withdrawn because of a terminal condition. More than two patients expiring in a week would be atypical.

On any given night during the pandemic, the trauma surgeon would continually walk around, managing over one hundred patients. Each of the four or five ICUs we covered was staffed with a team of nurses of varying experience, surgical residents, some volunteering general surgeons, and a member of our expert critical care physician assistant group. Our job was to manage all these sick patients like a central computer. Other surgical services chipped in to perform needed procedures. Because patient family members were not allowed to visit their ill relatives, the critical care team spent a large amount of time every day calling to give condition updates. Fortunately, by the summer, the number of patients had diminished to a fraction of the number treated in the spring, but the death toll was immense.

Long before COVID-19, before HIV/AIDS reared its ugly head in the early 1980s, the real killer from infection was—and is—hepatitis C. Until the last decade, there was no effective treatment for hepatitis C, which is transmitted by blood or fluid exchange. Hep C has caused cirrhosis of the liver in an enormous number of people (primarily baby boomers), and 25 percent of them developed chronic active hepatitis (which can kill a person without a liver transplant). According to the CDC, hepatitis C is the leading killer from infection in the United States today after COVID-19. Deaths associated with hepatitis C reached an all-time yearly high of 19,659 in 2014.

As a senior medical student, I was asked to come to the hospital ER and draw a blood sample from a Preludin addict who was as yellow as a highlighter (deep jaundice) from liver dysfunction. Preludin was a type of amphetamine (phenmetrazine) that was injected and could destroy a person's veins. No one could get any blood from this patient, so I used a tiny needle to get into the vein. Success! Then, as I filled the laboratory tube with blood, the needle flexed in the rubber stopper and came out the side, pricking my thumb. Blood welled up, and I remember anxiously thinking, "I'm gonna die." I ran over to my friend, the senior medical resident, who immediately went to get some immunoglobulin (all that we had in those days to try to prevent hepatitis). But when he injected me with the drug, he gasped and acted like he had used the wrong medication. Then he laughed and said, "Just kidding." I got a little light-headed, which was a first. After that experience, I experienced a vasovagal reaction with every shot, which means my heart rate drops to about zero, and I start to pass out. This uncontrollable physiological reaction has continued to occur for over forty years.

Later, as an intern, I learned the hard way why two shots are sometimes better than one. I was again asked to draw blood from a difficult patient. And for the second (and last) time, I managed to jab my finger with a "live" needle that had already been used to draw blood. (Fortunately, we now use a system that no longer requires us to push a thin needle through a rubber stopper.) This time, the patient had active syphilis. Seriously! So I marched down to the health clinic to get a shot of penicillin. Normally, the enormous dose of penicillin is split into two sizable doses, one for each buttock. I asked the nurse why I could not get just one dose in one ass cheek. She unfortunately complied, and I could not sit down for the next week. I had a golf ball–sized fluid collection of the antibiotic sitting in my derriere. Brilliant.

> **The human body is the only machine for which there are no spare parts.**
>
> HERMANN M. BIGGS (1859–1923)

The medical examiner showed us photos of the inside of the deceased's lungs. They were filled with a whitish substance that was identified as brain matter. The man had been standing behind an eighteen-wheeler truck that had slipped out of gear and rolled back, crushing him into a loading dock. The back of the truck had compressed the dead man's head almost flat, causing his brains to squirt down into his lungs through his trachea.

As I have gained seniority, I have begun to spend a small part of my time involved in legal work. For many years, I did consultation work for an organization that provided hospitals with "expert" opinions regarding their physicians' quality of care. My job was to comment on the appropriateness of trauma or surgical care, often after some poor patient outcomes, and to recommend some education or intervention. Over the years, I have been asked to function as an expert witness for physician defendants and on behalf of patient plaintiffs.

Recently, I reviewed the cases of patients who died suddenly to determine if they had any period of wakefulness before their demise. If you are maimed on a worksite and disabled, you and your family can receive lifelong financial support. But if you die, you are worth little; think two-thirds of your weekly salary for some time period based on your estimated years of productivity lost. (The recent Netflix movie *Worth* addressed this issue as it occurred among family members of those individuals who died on September 11.) But if the deceased experienced mental anguish before their death, that might warrant additional compensation for the surviving family members. On several occasions, I have been asked to adjudicate how long a person may have been awake (and potentially experienced pain or discomfort) before their last heartbeat. It usually just comes down to whether a prehospital provider or passerby noticed any sign of life and when those vital signs disappeared.

Trauma surgeons work closely with the medical examiner (ME) to understand the cause of death in situations where it is not obvious. Some years ago, I worked at a trauma center that was directly across the street from the ME's office, and we had an essentially 100 percent autopsy rate, meaning that all of the patients who died were examined by the ME to determine the cause of death. When there was a major question, because of our proximity to the

ME's office, we could send a surgeon or their designee over to watch the autopsy. At one point, we did a study to determine how often we missed any injury or condition that could have improved patient outcomes. Happily, we did not find any major omissions, probably because of the extensive imaging our patients undergo and the aggressiveness of our evaluations.

But the ME brings a different perspective, and it is helpful for us to hear from members of that office regularly, to better understand the injuries some of our patients sustained that led to their demise. The ME provides us with not only the cause of death but also the number of trauma deaths that never make it to the hospital, which is about 50 percent of all trauma-related deaths. Only when we have the full picture can we understand what changes need to occur in our homes, workplaces, and roadways to prevent injury.

The medical examiner presented slides of a pickup truck that had crashed next to an airport runway. We could see a plane landing through the front windshield from behind the vehicle where the deceased had probably looked up. He had lost control of the vehicle, crashing into a stationary object, and he had hurtled into the dashboard. As we moved closer, we could see where the man's head had struck the glass of the windscreen, and the top of his skull was missing. Then we were shown a photo of a trail of liquid (no doubt composed of cerebral spinal fluid and blood) on the roadway about 25 feet in front of the vehicle. This led up to the final resting place of the man's intact brain. I imagine that a person experiencing this type of injury would be unlikely to have any period of wakefulness that would warrant damages for potential mental anguish.

9

THE OPERATING THEATER

One of my surgical giant friends had in his operating room a
sign "If the operation is difficult, you aren't doing it right."
JOSEPH MURRAY (1919–2012),
WINNER OF THE NOBEL PRIZE IN MEDICINE

As a resident, I learned to go with the flow in the operating room. There
are all kinds of weird relationships between the OR staff and the sur-
geons. Some surgeons in the old days, like during my residency when
almost all the surgeons were men, had personal scrubs (people who hand
out instruments in the operating room). Today, there is a much higher
percentage of women surgeons (20 percent of general surgeons in 2015,
per the Association of American Medical Colleges, and women make up
half of some surgical residency programs). Back to personal scrub nurses,
these were typically very sharp, very highly skilled women who provided
superb support for the surgeons. As a student, I had a chance to rotate
with one of the leading vascular surgeons in the world. He would not
speak to his operating room nurse other than chitchat but would just put
out his open hand, and she would know what instrument he needed. In

one instance, he wanted something different than usual. The scrub nurse put about ten other instruments in his hand, one at a time, for about thirty seconds until he closed his hand over the correct instrument. That operating room was like a symphony, and it helped explain the exceptional results that the surgeon obtained.

One of the strangest operating room nurses was known as "Mary self-service." Working at a community hospital the residents called "the Carnage," Mary was a senior OR nurse (not a private scrub) who simply refused to do her job. We would have to assign an extra surgical resident, or sometimes the actual attending surgeon, to hand out the instruments. When she was asked why she refused to help on a case (as was her job), Mary would retort from the back of the OR where she would gab with the circulating nurse for the entire case, "You know I have been here for thirty-five years, and I will be retiring soon." It could not come too quickly for us.

Some surgeons prefer to cut in silence when they operate, but I like a variety of tunes. When I first walk into the operating room, I check on the age group of the OR staff. If everyone is nearing retirement, I select Sinatra or Marvin Gaye, or some oldie. I put on Dua Lipa or Gorillaz if the group is young. In between, there is funk, hip-hop, and reggae. I like to operate with music, with a few exceptions, usually cranked up to moderate decibels. It tends to make for a festive atmosphere, and the team is generally happy.

While writing this book, I walked into an operating room where one of my surgical residents, who I thought was about to assist me, was prepping a patient for surgery. I turned off the OR radio, put down my little Bluetooth speaker, and cranked up the tunes. Suddenly, everyone in the room was looking at me like I was crazy. I had barged into the wrong room (mine was next door) and turned off another surgeon's music. She was superfriendly about it. After profuse apologies from me and lots of laughter, I had some new friends.

> *The advent of anesthesia has made it so*
> *that any idiot can become a surgeon.*
>
> WILLIAM STEWART HALSTEAD (1852–1922)

After transport from a high-speed car crash scene, the woman's heart stopped as she arrived at the trauma center. We opened her chest, restarted her heart, and headed to the operating room. Restarting a heart is rare after blunt trauma, as it is hard to restore circulation when the heart stops as a result of blood loss. The "anesthesia A team" was in the operating room. Our crackerjack anesthesiologists gave this woman with a horrific injury (she tore her main vein to her small intestine, the superior mesenteric vein, off the portal vein, the major blood vessel returning venous blood to the liver) over 150 units of blood in about one hour. We were able to get her off the table and then returned to the OR three times in the next twenty-four hours as we performed as much surgery as she would tolerate. A few days later, we could close her chest and ultimately her abdomen with a skin graft. A year later, she was back on her treadmill working out. This was only possible because she had superb anesthesia resuscitation.

There are about fifty-one thousand board-certified anesthesiologists and thirty-nine thousand certified nurse anesthetists in the United States today. These folks put you to sleep and make sure you wake up. There are many specializations within the field, with anesthesiologists focusing on areas including pain, obstetrics, pediatrics, cardiac, neuroanesthesia, and critical care. Like surgical subspecialties, there are different personalities associated with the anesthesiology areas of expertise. For example, different competencies are required to care for a baby during surgery than are needed for an older adult's heart operation. In trauma, we often work closely with anesthesiology critical care folks. They are our brothers- and sisters-in-arms in both the surgical intensive care unit and in challenging trauma cases. There is nothing better than looking up in the operating room and seeing a highly competent anesthesia critical care colleague working with you in the treatment of a trauma patient. They are comfortable dealing with the most serious cases.

Anesthesiologists must work closely with surgeons if the patients are critically ill. I always say to surgical trainees that when they battle for the survival of a dying trauma patient, they need to be looking into the anesthesiologist's eyes "as if you're making love." Surgeons and anesthesiologists must work closely together if the patients are critically ill.

We often compress the aorta (main blood vessel to the abdomen) during bleeding trauma cases to allow our anesthesia colleagues to infuse blood and blood products. When the patient's blood volume is improved, we can feel this through the improved pulsations in the blood vessel. Then we can reduce our pressure and try to quickly eradicate the bleeding source. Most laypeople don't realize that patients do not bleed when their blood pressure is low. We cannot stop bleeding that is not evident. Once the pressure rises, we are better able to find a source. During this time when there is more bleeding, the blood pressure drops again, and we press on the aorta again. The anesthesiologist's role in the treatment of a patient who is dying after trauma is twofold: to monitor the patient's vital signs and, at the same time, to infuse massive volumes of blood and blood products in concert with interventions by the surgical team. This process of resuscitation and occlusion alternating with hemorrhage control requires cooperation. When the anesthesiology "A" team is working, it's like a symphony, and the patients have an optimal chance for survival.

After an aborted abdominal procedure, we rolled into the recovery room with a patient. She had undergone an open liver biopsy of some tiny lumps on the surface of her liver before a planned gastrectomy (removal of most of her stomach) for lymphoma, a type of cancer. Earlier, we had to hang around in the OR for over an hour telling jokes while we waited for a pathology report on the liver biopsy. We later aborted the operation (without performing the gastrectomy) when the expert team of pathologists and gastroenterologists could not agree on the type of lymphoma (therefore requiring a full pathologic evaluation, which typically requires a week to complete) and whether we should perform more radical surgery. In the recovery room, she woke up faster than anyone I had ever seen. I even mentioned this to my surgical team at the time. I circled back to the recovery room a few hours later to find a very anxious, upset patient. She said, "I remember that entire operation. I was awake the entire time." I responded that some folks felt they were awake, but I am sure it was just some of the medications. "No," she retorted. "I remember everything." And then she proceeded to relate to me two jokes I had told to everyone while we were waiting for the pathology results. She was alert and felt every part of the procedure but was paralyzed and unable to move. It is unclear how much pain she experienced. As awful as this sounds, it got even worse. A week later, the final pathology confirmed that this was the type of tumor that would require another operation to remove her stomach. The reluctant patient agreed only after we promised she would have a different anesthesiologist. Fortunately, only about one out of one thousand operations under general anesthesia are reported to result in "anesthesia awareness." I believe it must be a much rarer occurrence, as I have done many thousands of operations and only had this one case of anesthesia awareness.

Sometimes anesthesia can inadvertently impact the surgeon rather than the patient. One of my colleagues told me about the experience he had as a senior resident when performing a lung resection with a thoracic (chest) surgeon. During the operation, he kept dropping instruments and getting dizzy. This happened repeatedly during the case, to the consternation of the surgical faculty member, until they realized that it was occurring at a particular time during the operation when the bronchus was opened. This is the part of the lung anatomy that is connected to the trachea, where anesthetic gasses were being pumped into the patient. Basically, the senior resident was undergoing anesthesia without his knowledge. I guess sometimes we need to operate in scuba gear with an oxygen tank.

> *When I was young, patients were afraid of me; now that*
> *I am old, I am afraid of the patients.*
>
> JOHANN PETER FRANK (1745–1821)

As a resident, I occasionally rotated at community hospitals where there was quite a range of surgeon quality. The best operator was Dr. S, a superb general and vascular surgeon who was height-challenged and had a bit of a Napoleon complex. He was known as a perfectionist and a monster. My first exposure to Dr. S was as a floating second-year surgical

resident (the float resident was assigned to cover vacations for the first-
and second-year surgical residents throughout the various hospitals in our
training program, typically a week at a time). It was my first day there,
and I was sent by the chief resident into Dr. S's operating room, like a
lamb to the slaughter. As I entered the operating theater, Dr. S was melt-
ing down, screaming at the top of his lungs. His regular scrub nurse of
many years, Mrs. L, could take no more abuse. "F--- you, Dr. S!" she
shouted. The room became quiet. "I'd bet you would like to, Mrs. L,"
responded Dr. S. Everyone laughed, and the case went smoothly.

As a resident, I saw some bizarre surgeon behavior. I had just finished an inguinal hernia operation with Dr. C, which went well. I
was new to the hospital, and I thought the nurses were kidding me
when they asked me to stand in the corner of the operating room.
Dr. C then created a little circle of towels around the wound,
draped with sticky plastic material. The patient was rolled to their
side over a large plastic garbage can. Then Dr. C threw buckets
full of irrigation fluid (many gallons) at the wound, which splashed
off and ricocheted into the garbage can. When this ritual was
completed, I was allowed to close the skin. Dr. C was quite an
excellent surgeon, but his time operating in Vietnam had convinced him of the truth of the adage "the solution to pollution is
dilution," or, lots of irrigation was necessary to prevent wound
infections. (Actually, high-volume irrigation has been shown to
have no beneficial impact on infections.) The anesthesiologist told
me after the case that in the past, Dr. C had shorted out all the
anesthesia machines with his torrential waterfall of irrigation and
that the towel arrangement was the solution that the operating
room staff had devised.

Our surgical chairman, "Lester," was a physically large man who was a brilliant surgeon. While doing a case with Lester, he would recite entire textbooks' worth of information on surgical anatomy, history, and physiology while expecting you to absorb all the data and continue operating. I wish I had recorded all the information he imparted, as it was easy to be overwhelmed by the volume of data when concentrating on performing a complex procedure. If you slowed down to listen to his dialogue or leaned forward into his field of vision, he would coldcock you with his forehead. I remember being smacked only once and seeing stars for a while afterward. To keep the resident from dawdling, he would not let them use scissors, so all the dissection occurred exclusively with the scalpel. I remember resecting a pancreatic pseudocyst from its location between the duodenum and the inferior vena cava (the surgeons reading this will get chills now . . . this is a complicated and treacherous procedure) exclusively with a scalpel. But we got good with the knife. We used to say that the chairman could take an intern through a hepatectomy (guide a junior surgical resident through a complex surgery); he was that superb. The most charismatic surgeon in our training program was the residency program director, Dr. D (who, not surprisingly, went on to become a chair of surgery and a medical school dean). As a senior resident running his vast surgical oncology service, I asked Dr. D for permission to have his favorite psychiatrist consult one of his patients. He responded, "The psychiatrist should see me and all of my patients daily."

The residents and faculty identified some surgeons as poor or downright unsafe technicians. One of my surgical interns told me of his experiences during medical school in New Orleans with a notorious surgeon nicknamed HODAD (this stood for "hands of death and destruction"). These characters were out there, but they were well known. When I arrived as chief resident at one community hospital, I was summoned to the office of the chief of surgery and informed that a particular surgeon (whom all the residents referred to as Dr. Blown-apart) was not to operate on anyone without either the senior resident or me in the room to "assist." This surgeon was very old and past his prime. But it was not always the old guys who were the problems. I should be clear that most senior surgeons have a tremendous amount of wisdom, and it is a shame when they retire and take all that experience and the associated battle scars with them. I used to tell the older members of my department years later that they could die, but they were not allowed to retire. Their perspective, experience, and intuition were irreplaceable, even if they had a lot of peculiarities.

Of course, idiosyncrasies are not the exclusive province of surgeons. During my residency years at a community hospital, a cardiologist, the head of the cardiac care unit (CCU), was admitted with chest pain to his own ICU. He was a morbidly obese middle-aged man built like a large penguin. The CCU was shaped in a crescent around the nursing station, with large glass walls and sliding glass doors for each room, so the nurses could easily see the patients and their heart monitors. In the middle of the night, a patient had a cardiac arrest. The CCU director got out of his hospital bed and, in his flimsy gown (with his huge derriere hanging out the back), went to the coding patient's bedside and ran the code blue. This was easily visible to all the other patients in the CCU, who then experienced their own crushing chest pain at the sight of a half-naked patient running a medical code in front of them.

Freedom is the oxygen of the soul.

Moshe Dayan (1915–1981)

Decades ago, I got to experience the effects of reduced oxygen on my tissues. No, I did not attempt to summit Mt. Everest. It was nothing that grand or ambitious. The problem began when I made the mistake of mixing aerobic workouts on a stationary rower with a highly competitive tennis game, after which I developed "golfer's elbow." This inflammation of the medial (inside) aspect of the elbow is commonly associated with golf (which I don't play), and it became a nagging and painful problem. It got to the point that, during a tennis match, I needed to carry my racket to the net in my unaffected hand while I waited to have sensation return in the arm that had just served the ball.

Finally, after the failure of multiple other nonsurgical remedies (including steroid injections) over a two-year period, my hand surgeon agreed to operate on my elbow. But the first available time she had was the afternoon before I was scheduled for a night of trauma call. I made the anesthesiologist promise to avoid anesthesia or sedation (as I needed my faculties to operate a few hours later), and they completed the procedure. I miscalculated by thinking that local anesthetics would take care of any discomfort I would experience. For an operation on the elbow, the surgeons use a special tourniquet. This eliminates blood loss by cutting off all the circulation to the extremity. But it also induces the most severe ischemia (when no oxygen is getting to the tissues). Usually, the patient is under general anesthesia and does not feel anything, but I spent the half-hour procedure biting down on a rag (think gnawing on a leather belt during an amputation in the Wild West) while I got to experience my own little childbirth-level pain. When the tourniquet was turned off and my circulation was restored, it felt like a cool river flowed down my arm, and I had a moment of euphoria. I felt like I had been tortured (albeit self-induced). I should state that the operation was an immediate success.

In our absolute need for oxygen, we are no different from the one-celled organisms from which we evolved. The body plan of most multicellular organisms can be reduced to a simple scheme based on the delivery of oxygen to the tissues. Oxygen is poorly soluble in water and plasma; therefore, most multicellular organisms with a cardiovascular system have evolved a respiratory pigment that serves to bind and carry oxygen in the blood. In vertebrates (like humans), the respiratory pigment (always hemoglobin) is packaged in red blood cells.

Air was poorly understood until the late eighteenth century, when Carl Wilhelm Scheele, a Swedish chemist, and Joseph Priestley, an English minister and amateur chemist, independently discovered oxygen. Priestley lived next to a brewery and became fascinated by the immense quantities of gas that were bubbling up in the brewing vats, in which a candle could not burn. He began performing experiments with gases. Priestley went on to discover nine new gases, refrigeration, soda water, and oxygen generation by photosynthesis (the process by which green plants use sunlight to synthesize foods from carbon dioxide and water to produce oxygen). It is well known that our current monitoring techniques of systemic parameters (such as heart rate and blood pressure) do not identify regional ischemia in essential organs, so we often underestimate how sick our trauma patients are. Some years ago, we started investigating the value of near-infrared spectroscopy to assess trauma patients to diagnose "shock" or hypoperfusion (inadequate oxygen delivery) of the tissues. Near-infrared spectroscopy assesses venous blood hemoglobin saturation, which, along with capillary blood, makes up 90 percent of the blood volume in tissues. Near-infrared spectroscopy permits continuous, noninvasive measurement of tissue hemoglobin oxygen saturation in muscle. A few years ago, working with colleagues across the country, we showed that these noninvasive probes provided information about oxygen saturation in the tissues of trauma patients, which was as valuable as pulse and blood pressure in predicting who is in shock from bleeding. Therefore, we can measure the oxygen in body tissues using a probe lying on the skin's surface. Think of a "tricorder" from the Star Trek TV series (a futuristic device that supposedly measured body chemistry and physiology).

The reputation of a surgeon, in the final analysis,
must rest upon: originality; teaching by word of mouth; teaching
by the printed word; and operative skill.

WILLIAM J. MAYO (1861–1939)

The surgical fellow began the abdominal exploration and was exposing the surgical field for the repair of an abdominal aortic aneurysm. The famous cardiovascular surgeon then scrubbed into the case. "Sir, your hands are in my field of vision," he said. The fellow responded unwisely, "Gee, Dr. DeBakey, I thought you could see through anything." The retort came quickly: "Sir, I can see through your head, but I cannot see through your hands." Recognize that Dr. Michael DeBakey basically invented this operation and was known to devour residents and fellows like BBQ ribs. This fellow, David Feliciano, survived and went on to become a leading trauma surgeon in the United States.

During my career, I had several opportunities to get to know some giants in the field. One of the first giants, and a true gentleman, was Dr. Denton Cooley, one of the world's great cardiac surgeons and a true surgical innovator. When I was an intern, I visited him with one of his cardiologists in his office. I was stunned that Dr. Cooley took the time to meet me and make me feel like the only person in the room. Here was one of the leading surgeons in the world, whose book I had recently read as a student, focusing on a lowly junior resident. Years later, as a surgical leader, I had the pleasure of inviting Denton to be our visiting professor, which he graciously accepted on several occasions.

Stanley Dudrick was another giant I got to know quite well in my role as a monthly visiting surgical educator for his residency program. He was another true gentleman. As a resident, Dr. Dudrick led the efforts to develop total parenteral nutrition, a complete intravenous nutritional diet, which has subsequently been used to sustain countless patients when they could not eat for prolonged periods. Along with preparing the intravenous food solutions, Stan had to develop methods of vascular access. He also helped devise strategies to insert the special intravenous catheters that can remain in the vein for extended periods. As a resident at a national conference, he famously showed two beagle puppies that grew to be healthy adult dogs, one consuming puppy chow and the other subsisting on a diet exclusively of intravenous nutrients. Total parenteral nutrition is now a routine part of medical care and has saved innumerable lives worldwide. Stan helped open the doors for me to move to one of my most important trauma positions.

I also had the opportunity to work with Basil Pruitt for several years. One of the world's leading surgical researchers and burn surgeons, Dr. Pruitt was responsible for dramatically lowering mortality rates from burns. The risk of death from burns correlates with the percent of skin injured of the total body surface area (TBSA) affected. In the 1950s, when Dr. Pruitt began to work in this field, the LD50 (the burn size resulting in death 50 percent of the time) for thermal injuries was about 42 percent. Over Dr. Pruitt's thirty-year career, the LD50 rose to more than 90 percent TBSA for burned patients. In addition, while at the US Army Institute of Surgical Research, Basil led both investigative and clinical efforts in burn care and trained many of the world's burn surgeons.

The surgical giant who made the most long-lasting impact on me was probably Claude Organ. Dr. Organ had been the chairman of surgery at a medical school in the Midwest and later in his career had moved to run a program in the San Francisco Bay Area. On a return flight from a visit to my parents with my children, I ran into Dr. Organ for the first and only time. I was trespassing in first class with my toddler son who could not wait another minute for the bathroom to become available in the economy section. Dr. Organ questioned me about my hat, which displayed the word "Trauma." We began an hour-long conversation that influenced my entire academic career. Dr. Organ told me a story of how he had operated on the president of a major corporation with excellent results. As a gesture of gratitude, this executive arranged for a personal leadership consultation for Dr. Organ. The organization sent a gentleman in an elegant three-piece suit to take detailed notes on Dr. Organ's management style. Dr. Organ, being the animated, loquacious character he was, could not wait for the written results and inquired of this efficiency expert: "How am

I doing?" The response was "I am sure you are a great surgeon, but as a manager, you're a disaster area."

Dr. Organ ran his business as I did at that time, as an office with an open door and zero time management. Dr. Organ related to me the recommendations that were made to him by these management experts, and I incorporated all of them into my hectic life. My productivity instantly improved exponentially. So, standing in the aisle of a flight across America, an hour of conversation with one man entirely changed my professional life.

These four men changed the surgical world, and it was an honor to get to know them. Sadly, they all passed away during the last decade, but each left a huge legacy.

10

ARE SURGEONS DANGEROUS?

*The pilot is by circumstances allowed only one serious mistake,
while the surgeon may commit many and not even
recognize his own errors as such.*
JOHN S. LOCKWOOD (1907–1950)

The senior resident informed me that an X-ray showed a foreign object (a large gauze or "lap" pad) in the belly. One of my young faculty partners, Dr. G, had taken out a young woman's diseased gallbladder and had accidentally left a gauze pad in the abdomen. Dr. G had left town on holiday, so now I was the covering surgeon. We took the patient back to the operating room and removed the lap pad after a thirty-minute procedure. The patient did well and had no residual effect. Later, she sued Dr. G and the hospital for millions of dollars in a case that made the local paper's front page and included my partner's name. The day this was reported by the press, my same partner risked his life removing an unexploded live grenade embedded in a patient's abdomen who had arrived at the trauma center after a mishap at a local munitions plant. Retained foreign body cases (like the lap pad) are rare and were settled in those *days for around $75,000. But because of the enormous claim by the plaintiff, the case went to trial. The jury awarded the patient only about $25,000. Dr. G was so upset by the notoriety of having his name in the paper that he quit practicing surgery, obtained an MBA, and became a computer IT person.*

About fifteen hundred of some twenty-eight million surgeries performed each year in the United States result in a foreign body retained inside the patient. In each operation, surgeons make significant effort to avoid leaving any instruments or other objects behind at the surgical site. The large gauze pads that we use during abdominal operations and all the instruments are counted before and after any procedure. If the count is incorrect, we reexplore the entire operative site. Certain situations make retention of an instrument or lap pad more likely: if the case is an emergency, if it is particularly long and the OR support team changes, or if there is more than one group of operating surgeons (like general surgeons helping some gynecologists). If there is any concern about the count or if something may be missing, we obtain a set of X-rays. Today, in the rare circumstance when a foreign body is retained, the hospital will typically pay for all medical expenses and settle for around $100,000. How quickly we diagnose the presence of a retained foreign body and any complications that result are essential in determining the financial costs.

Why was this man craning his neck to the left side? "Mr. O, why are you looking to the side?" we asked the older man after a car crash. "Does it hurt?" we wondered. "No, it feels better this way," he responded. Naturally, we were concerned that Mr. O had a broken neck. We did all types of imaging, and the diagnosis (in the days before MRI) was that he had torticollis, a bad muscle spasm. Subsequently, we did physical therapy work with him to get some movement in his neck. We found him craning his neck to the right (opposite) side a few days later. We again asked Mr. O, "Why are you looking to that side?" "Feels better this way," he stated again. We repeated every imaging study, and all were reread as normal. As the physical therapists attempted to mobilize his neck again for torticollis, the radiologist most expert in cervical spine imaging returned from vacation. He immediately diagnosed the patient with a condition called "jumped facets." The stabilizing ligaments of his spine were disrupted, and the broken bones of his cervical spine were locked into position. A wrong move could have caused him to be permanently paralyzed. We were unsure how all the spine surgery experts and radiologists had missed this finding and how the physical therapy had not resulted in further injury. But we had the opportunity to revisit images of his injuries daily, as wall-sized photos were displayed on a poster at the entry of the radiology department. Every time we walked by, we shuddered to think how close we had come to making this man a quadriplegic by causing a spinal cord injury.

Where No Man Has Gone Before.

STAR TREK MOTTO

I was walking by the OR late one morning when the door to the OR suite swung open, and from the end of the hall, someone yelled for me to help them immediately. I was already in scrubs, so I donned a surgical cap and mask and ran into the room. The orthopedists had been inserting some hardware into a middle-aged woman with a broken femur. She had arrived earlier after a car crash when she had a sudden drop in her end-tidal CO_2 *(exhaled carbon dioxide concentration). This signifies something very terrible going on with the circulation (think of something blocking the bloodstream or the heart stopping). In this case, we suspected the cause was a pulmonary embolism (a big blood clot in the lung circulation). The very experienced and knowledgeable chief of trauma anesthesiology, Dr. V, told me that a catastrophe had occurred, and I believed him. So I attempted a rarely performed procedure called a pulmonary embolectomy for the first time. I was twenty years out of medical school and had never even seen this operation done, ever. It is always challenging to do an operation you have only read about. Huge clots to the lung circulation can be fatal and are fortunately exceedingly rare, but this situation of near cardiac arrest suggested the diagnosis. In fact, 50 percent of people with massive pulmonary emboli die within thirty minutes. (Usually, clots to the lung are tiny blobs called microemboli that cause abnormal lung function by stimulating the release of specific chemicals leading to constriction of the lung tissue and its blood supply and poor oxygen levels in the blood. But the microemboli do not make you have a catastrophic presentation of near death, typically.)*

There was no time to watch a YouTube video or call a senior consultant. I was there; she was dying, and I had to act. I performed a sternotomy (opening the middle of the chest to expose the heart), which was the easy part. I then isolated and opened the pulmonary artery; we removed a massive clot. At about that time, one of the cardiothoracic surgeons arrived, but it was too late. Unfortunately, the patient's heart had stopped beating just as we entered the chest. Even after placing her on cardiopulmonary bypass, we were unsuccessful in getting her heart restarted. In retrospect, the diagnosis was correct, and we did everything about as quickly and expeditiously as possible, but sometimes the insult is beyond our ability to correct. Having to perform any procedure for the first time on a dying patient is entering unfamiliar territory without much of a map, à la Lewis and Clark. But a surgeon is expected to be ready to deal with adversity and be nimble, as an operative case occasionally requires a considerable amount of ingenuity or, as we say, "making do."

> *If a meteor strikes you, that is an act of God,*
> *and you can consider it an "accident." Otherwise,*
> *injuries are probably avoidable.*
>
> STEPHEN M. COHN, M.D.

The man was sitting in the barber chair, getting a trim. Next door, workers were renovating a commercial space. One of them was using a nail gun to mount some paneling when he missed the stud and shot a nail through the wall, striking the barber's customer in the neck and severing his spinal cord. Just like that, he was quadriplegic for life. It turns out that nail guns are potentially very lethal. They employ a charge sufficient to drive huge nails into concrete. Some years ago, we devised an animal model to study blasts to the torso. (Subsequently, this allowed us to make observations that helped us save human lives.) We wanted to replicate a previous animal model that used blanks from a handgun to induce a shock wave. But there was simply no way to use and store a gun in the medical center. We thought of using a nail gun to induce an injury via a metal disc placed on the torso of an anesthetized pig. The hardware store sent over a technician to train us amateurs in using the nail gun. "There are four possible charges we could use," the expert informed us. "We will start with the lowest charge." (This charge had the power of a .22 handgun, in the form of a blank.) The blank explodes and drives a metal plunger out the end of the nail gun into the metal disc. In our animal, this initial charge appeared to work effectively. We then clamored to try the number 4 (highest) power charge. The technician squinted at us as if we were excitable teenagers and said, "We will try the number two charge." He had us back away from the animal and watch. When the nail gun fired, the metal disc exploded through the pig and exited the other side of its torso, embedding in the wall about 6 feet away. He gazed at us stunned observers and said, "And that's why you will be using the lowest power charge."

One of the hardest things to deal with as a trauma team is the truly innocent person who is injured while minding their own business. It is easier to understand how trauma can occur when someone does something stupid, like driving under the influence or playing with guns. But when a random event strikes them down, it seems like an act of God. Therefore, we rarely use the term "accident." This implies there was nothing anyone could have done to avoid trauma. While texting is overemphasized as a cause of distracted driving, there are many other types of avoidable distracting behavior: eating while driving, changing the radio station while driving, or whacking your misbehaving kids in the back seat while driving. But we do occasionally see a patient with an injury from an incident that appears unavoidable. I remember a woman who arrived at the trauma center shaking but uninjured after a bad car crash. She was a passenger in the front seat of a car commuting to work. A huge truck tire became dislodged from an eighteen-wheeler heading in the opposite direction on the highway and bounced over the cement dividers. The tire had dropped through the car's roof, killing the driver instantly. We made sure this patient received access to counseling to help her deal with this horrible experience.

Technical difficulties are rarely insurmountable with practice,
ingenuity, and the passage of time.

ELLIOTT CARR CUTLER (1888–1947)

Recently, I watched a documentary describing how a group of Nepalese climbers scaled the fourteen highest peaks in the world, all over 8,000 meters high, in seven months. The toughest of these peaks is K2, where 25 percent of people who attempted the climb have died, and, as of 2021, only 377 people have summited and lived to talk about it (more earthlings have traveled to outer space). If you think four hundred summiting K2 sounds like a lot of people, by comparison, more than ten thousand people have successfully climbed Mt. Everest.

The K2 for trauma surgeons is probably a blunt retrohepatic vena cava injury. This huge vein runs up to the heart from behind the liver. Many surgeons have never had a patient survive this type of damage. (I am fortunate enough to have had a few.) There are multiple issues with the repair of this injury; the first is that the patients are very unstable due to blood loss and the abdomen is entirely full of blood. One suspects this is a potential injury when blood gushes (audible bleeding) from behind the liver when there is no upward pressure exerted by the surgeon. Because of the location and the fact that this is the primary venous blood return to the heart, if you apply too much pressure, you limit the blood filling the heart and the patient becomes hypotensive (low blood pressure). But if you don't apply enough pressure, more bleeding occurs and you are flooded with blood. This leaves the surgeon between the proverbial rock and a hard place. The second issue is the exposure of the injury, as this is an exceedingly difficult area of the abdomen to reveal, requiring a couple of incisions. We have learned from our liver transplant colleagues that extending our up-and-down midline incision to the upper-right part of the abdomen (called "T-ing off the incision") allows us to see the injury once the liver is rolled over. The third issue is that anesthesia needs to have access to a lot of blood for transfusion and must be able to function independently in maintaining resuscitation. We partially compress the aorta for these procedures, but the right amount of blood and blood products must be given, or we are utterly underwater without scuba gear. Finally, once the injury is exposed, we need to quickly place a set of clamps on the defect and suture it closed. This requires an experienced surgeon to use their hands to expose the area and guide the other surgeon to do the repair. Many things have to go smoothly for a person to survive this most severe "K2" of all injuries.

The safest thing for a patient is to be in the hands of a man engaged in teaching medicine. In order to be a teacher of medicine the doctor must always be a student.

CHARLES H. MAYO (1865–1939)

After a medical conference, an orthopedist, a plastic surgeon, and a general surgeon were captured by terrorist forces. They were informed late in the evening that negotiations had broken down and they were to be executed at dawn. They were told that, as was their custom, their captors would grant one reasonable request to each of them. The orthopedic surgeon said that he was quite an epicure, so he would enjoy a multicourse Middle Eastern feast as his last wish. The plastic surgeon stated that he would like to give one more lengthy presentation with dual projectors of all his favorite before and after cosmetic slides. After hearing he would be subjected to the plastic surgeon's soliloquy, the general surgeon said, "You can kill me now."

In the late 1990s, my colleagues and I expanded a large fellowship program in trauma and surgical critical care in Florida. We made a concerted effort to recruit the best and brightest surgical trainees from North America and invited surgeons worldwide. For whatever reason, we found ourselves with several excellent surgical fellows from Israel and other countries in the Middle East (Lebanon, Saudi Arabia, and Egypt). The international fellows were great personalities and all got along famously. You would never know that their nations were sworn enemies.

For a while, many of the trauma centers in Israel were led by my former fellows. When I visited Israel for a surgical conference, they would arrange a casual dinner at one of their homes in Tel Aviv. We would have a grand time reminiscing. Of course, with all of us sitting by the BBQ at one table for dinner, one random missile could have severely damaged the Israeli trauma leadership.

One of my fellows was from Okinawa. Dr. M sat quietly, observing all the hospital antics for quite some time. He rarely spoke. I frankly did not know what to make of him. Suddenly, after about six months, he started to talk to us and revealed that he was brilliant and downright hilarious. I have had the pleasure of training thousands of students and residents and over one hundred fellows. Many of my former fellows are senior surgeons now, running residency programs, trauma services, surgical ICUs, and, in some instances, entire surgery departments. I have learned something from working with each of them. To be clear, helping individuals become mature, capable surgeons is undoubtedly, along with caring for patients, the most rewarding aspect of my surgical career.

11

FRIENDS IN THE TRAUMA TRENCHES

HOW MY NIECE'S MISERABLE DRIVING
SKILLS SAVED A LIFE
By Yoram Klein, M.D.

Lindsey is my beloved niece. She is a bright, beautiful young real estate agent. She has many fine qualities. Driving skills were never one of them. If car insurance agents had kept a secret blacklist, Lindsey would have been the star of it. Therefore, I wasn't surprised when my brother-in-law called me one afternoon and said that Lindsey had had a severe motor vehicle collision and the ambulance was taking her to the trauma center where I was working. She had apparently left the highway in a busy interchange, taken a wrong turn, and driven into oncoming traffic . . . a few seconds later, the inevitable head-on collision happened. The other driver, Mary, was also rushed to my center. She was one of the most admirable patients I ever treated. Very calm, cooperative, and patient. Her main concern was Lindsey's condition. She kept asking us about how she felt and her general condition. She even talked with Lindsey across the curtain that separated the two beds, calming and reassuring her that everything was okay.

Lindsey was alert, with normal breathing and blood pressure, but she was complaining about everything—a condition that, in Israel, we call KBS, or Kula Buga syndrome (*kula buga* in Arabic means "everything is painful"). I always told her parents that they spoiled her too much. . . . The total body CT scan was normal except for a minor fracture of the pubic bone in the pelvis, which did not need any intervention except for some pain medication.

Mary's CT scan, on the other hand, revealed a large traumatic abdominal wall hernia with bowel loops under the skin of the left flank. So we admitted her to the trauma step-down unit for observation and planned to reconstruct her abdominal wall in a delayed fashion if everything went smoothly. Five minutes later, an urgent call arrived from the attending radiologist. He reexamined the CT scan and found a large tumor inside Mary's heart. Had it not been detected, this tumor could have caused catastrophic complications. Three days later, Mary had an open-heart operation, and the cancer was successfully removed. She recovered, and, three months later, we reconstructed her abdominal wall. After a short recovery, Mary went back to her everyday life. That was the first time in my career that I heard a trauma victim refer to the person who caused her injury as "my guardian angel."

BROKEN HEARTS AND SPLEENS
By Dror Soffer, M.D.

It was a dark, rainy night in Tel Aviv when my phone woke me up. The EMS on the phone announced an MVC (motor vehicle crash):

a forty-year-old woman, a safety belt injury, abdominal and chest pain, stable, ETA ten minutes. I put on my scrubs and took the elevator to the ER floor. My fingers knew the code on the door to the trauma room by heart. The sliding doors opened, and I glided inside, waking up with every step I made. My trauma team was already there waiting for the victim to arrive. Soon enough, after donning the protective gear, I nodded to my chief resident and heard the automatic announcement system: "Trauma team to the trauma bay." The front doors opened, and the EMS team carried a woman inside. "She lost control in the rain, and the car was thrown to the side of the road and hit a tree. We found her outside in a ditch . . ." the report went on as the patient was transferred to the trauma stretcher. The residents and nurses started with the primary survey routine, and as I supervised their actions, I was fascinated by the woman's face. She was lovely, but I could not ignore her pale face and fast breathing. Her eyes were mahogany brown, and she was quietly crying. When Boaz, the chief resident, asked her, "Where does it hurt, ma'am?" she kept silent but pointed with her right hand to her chest. She looked stable enough, apart from the seat belt sign (a linear band-like bruise across the abdomen or chest resulting from the force induced by the restraint device).

We decided to scan her, as we were impressed by the mechanism of injury and the seat belt sign. The CT scan showed a minor laceration of the spleen, so we admitted her for observation. Just before leaving the trauma bay, I got a phone call. "She keeps complaining of chest pain, and her ECG shows signs of acute myocardial infarction," said the resident. I rushed back inside. What could it be? An acute coronary event? Blunt cardiac injury? We consulted the cardiologists, who agreed to perform an urgent cardiac catheterization to rule out an acute cardiac event. In this procedure, some anticoagulants might be involved and could cause intra-abdominal bleeding, so we all went with her to the cath lab to be readily available for any catastrophe. I noticed that the patient was silently crying during the procedure. The heart catheterization was conclusive for takotsubo cardiomyopathy, also known as "broken heart syndrome." (This is a condition where the heart muscle becomes suddenly weakened, usually because of severe emotional or physical stress. Fortunately, it is reversible.[1]) When we told her the diagnosis, she suddenly stopped crying and said, "Amazing, you can see it in my heart; my husband and I separated three days ago, and the pain in my chest has been there ever since."

GUNSHOT WOUND FROM FROBISHER BAY
By Robert Chernak, M.D.

As the chief orthopedic resident at the Royal Victoria Hospital in Montreal, I assessed all trauma coming into the ER. McGill University Hospitals were the catchment areas for all the Quebec territories and the Arctic centers in Northern Canada. It was not unusual to have med flights coming in from the far reaches of Northern Canada with different types of trauma cases. So that evening, when I was informed of an incoming flight of a twenty-two-year-old male with a gunshot wound, it seemed relatively routine. When assessed in the ER, he had a normal blood pressure and pulse, but there was a small entrance wound in the belly button area. Once his entire assessment was complete and there was no orthopedic issue detected, he was handed over to the general surgical service for exploration of his abdomen.

As a detailed history was taken and he was asked about the nature of his injury, the young man was less than forthcoming with any significant details. His toxic screen was negative, and he was not on drugs or alcohol. Before my handoff to the other service, I went back and discussed his case with him. It was not unusual for young Inuit patients to be involved with knife and gun trauma, but those injuries were usually associated with a bar fight. I had developed a connection with this young man, and when we started to talk before his general surgical intervention, he described exactly what had happened. He said he had shot himself. I inquired if he wished to take his own life. He said no. On further questioning, he told me the absolute truth: "I was bored!" He admitted that he used a small-caliber weapon and not one of his big hunting rifles, assuming that he would get a med flight into Montreal to see something other than snow and ice and a large open ocean. He was a perfectly balanced young man except for his warped rationale about how to leave his Inuit village. But it certainly did redefine the term "bored" for me.

ONLY IN LA
By Gary Bellach, M.D.

Los Angeles is home to the film and television production industry. Film crews often employ facial moulage impressions: prosthetic sculpting, molding, and casting techniques to create advanced cosmetic effects. These techniques were first used in the 1902 movie *A Trip to the Moon* to make the man-on-the-moon effect. Other films that used these techniques were *Frankenstein* featuring Boris Karloff, *The Wolf Man*, and *Planet of the Apes*. These accurate impressions are created using prosthetic alginate, a naturally occurring polysaccharide found in brown algae that forms a viscous gum when hydrated. This alginate sets quickly after being poured into a hard mold jacket or matrix using plaster, fiberglass, and acrylic.

Late one afternoon, a film production technician presented to my ENT office with a rock-hard white acrylic "cast" filling the left nasal cavity. The flow of the fast-setting liquid is difficult to control once poured. In his case, the liquid was poured and had quickly set without adequate nasal protection, and it filled the entire nasal cavity. All the office procedures I tried to dislodge this "cast" failed.

Much later that evening, with the patient in the hospital operating room under general anesthesia, I used every device available on the standard nasal instrument tray—without success. At this point, the nurses in the operating room, the anesthesiologist, and the operating surgeon (me) were all wondering what to do. This prompted a very remote medical school memory from my orthopedic surgery rotation. The ENT surgeon had asked the nurses for an orthopedic bone instrument tray. This did little to instill confidence in the operating room team. "Why is this ENT guy failing with ENT instruments, asking for orthopedic equipment?"

Our team thus employed an orthopedic bone cutter (stainless steel Liston 7.5 inch) to successfully cut the rock-hard acrylic mass into multiple small fragments to facilitate complete removal. The surgeon's angina chest pain resolved. The technician's nose returned to normal. Only in LA!

IT IS NOT ABOUT YOU
By John Bini, M.D.

Father's Day 2007, Balad, Iraq

I woke up on Father's Day in 2007 in the desert halfway around the world. I was miserable. Father's Day—I was supposed to be with my family. I missed my family, and I missed my kids. Why was I here? I was feeling sorry for myself. It was just another hot, miserable, dusty day in the cradle of civilization. What is so civilized about people shooting and blowing each other up? To top it off, I was part of a planned army/air force surgeon swap and was going to fly in a frigging helicopter to Baghdad later that day. I would probably get shot at.

You never really have a day off in a combat zone. We started with the usual smattering of gunshot wounds and IED (improvised explosive device) blasts: nothing unusual, just a steady flow of carnage. War is unique in that she's not very selective about whom she affects: combatants, noncombatants, soldiers, sailors, marines, aircrew, NATO forces, Iraqi forces, good guys, bad guys (whatever that means), men, women, children, young and old. The macabre reality of war is that she's fair and does not discriminate when she doles out her death and devastation.

We were notified of some incoming traumas. A nearby village had been attacked. Two young Iraqi males arrived at the combat hospital, both with multiple torso injuries. I took one of them to the operating room, and one of my partners, TJ, took the other. TJ's patient was sick. TJ opened his chest in the operating room, and, despite heroic efforts, the patient died on the table. My patient seemed to be faring a little better, even though he had many bowel injuries and his liver needed to be packed (placement of large gauze pads to compress the liver and stop ongoing bleeding). Damage control in the belly was completed; the kid, however, had a penetrating head wound. He was cold and in shock. Instead of going to the head CT scan, I had our neurosurgeon (who was later shot and became a patient of mine . . . I told you war was fair) put in an ICP (intracranial pressure) monitor. My patient's intracranial pressure was equal to his mean arterial pressure (so he had little if any blood flow to his brain); his pupils were fixed and dilated. At about this time, we heard that his dad had arrived. We allowed the father and the lay clergy to come into the operating room and pray with the patient as he was dying. The father was distraught. As we tried to allow the patient to die with as much dignity as possible, we found out that the patient who died in TJ's OR was my patient's brother. The father, mourning the death of one son, was now watching his other son die within an hour—Father's Day in Iraq.

Fast-forward a few hours, and it was time to get on the helicopter and head to Baghdad. I packed my backpack and met my orthopedic colleague joining me for the trip, and we headed off to catch our flight. As we sat quietly waiting, the orthopedist asked me if I was okay. I lost it. I was crying hysterically. I felt so cheap, so superficial, so selfish. My babies were at home, safe, not getting shelled while playing soccer in the front yard. How could I have been so self-centered and full of self-pity earlier in the day? The lesson in this, I guess, is that it is not about me. It is about patients, their families, and the noble calling of medicine and surgery to serve and help others relieve pain and suffering. Father's Day has never been the same for me, but, more importantly, I have never been the same.

THE ONGOING CHALLENGE TO
OVERCOME MOTHER NATURE
By Alan Lisbon, M.D.

It's very unusual for an experienced ICU nurse to get rattled. They've seen many things, and nothing causes them to lose their cool or control. It was strange, then, for me to walk into the ICU to begin rounds and hear one of the senior nurses screaming from one of the patient rooms. I ran to the room and found the nurse up on a chair pointing at the patient and shrieking. The patient was a fifty-year-old man who'd had a Whipple procedure two days before. (This entails the removal of the first part of the intestine and most of the pancreas, a complex procedure.)

Coming out of the patient's nose was a large worm. The worm was about three-quarters of an inch in diameter, and 10 inches long. It crawled out of the patient's nose, landed on his hospital gown, and wiggled down to his abdomen where we grabbed it, put it in a jar of formalin, and sent it off to the pathologist. It turns out the worm was an *Ascaris lumbricoides* (roundworm). About a billion people in the world are infected with these worms. The eggs are found in dirt and water and are ingested when sanitary conditions are not so great. The eggs hatch in the small intestine, and the larvae then migrate through the intestinal wall into the bloodstream where they are brought to the liver and lungs. Once in the lungs, they crawl up the trachea and are ingested and mature in the gut. They can grow to between 15 and 35 centimeters long, and there can be multiple worms. Often, after surgery, they become restless and will migrate either toward the mouth or the rectum. They also have been known to come out of tear ducts, the umbilicus, or the inguinal region. Treatment with an antiparasitic like albendazole is highly effective. Our patient had come from Ecuador, where he had become infected, and the worms had decided to move out after anesthesia and surgery.

LISTEN TO THE PATIENT
By John Bini, M.D.

I've had the unique opportunity of being both a surgeon and a patient at the same institution . . . more than once. It was June, and I was ready to have a wonderful summer. My work schedule was set, and vacation plans were made. I was having a routine endoscopy as part of my annual health maintenance. In medical school, I was diagnosed with colon cancer, which was treated with surgery and chemotherapy. Since then, I have had an annual screening endoscopy. Early on, it was a very stressful time of year. I always worried about what they would find. Thankfully, I had made it twenty years without recurrence. The screening had become a rather routine, non-stress-provoking event.

So I was stunned when I woke up after my endoscopy to discover that my doctor had found an abnormal-looking lesion in my stomach. My GI doc told me that it just looked funny, and it hadn't been there last year, so he took a bunch of biopsies and said we'd wait and see what the pathologist said. All I could think about was my mortality, my wife, and my children. I was scared. All my medical knowledge did nothing to alleviate this anxiety and fear. The pathology results returned indeterminate, so I underwent another endoscopy, this time with a partial removal of the mass. This time, the diagnosis was gastric cancer.

I casually mentioned to my team the next day that I would be their patient. In many ways, this simple statement was the bridge for me from doctor to patient. It was a lot easier being the doctor. I had surgery to remove part of my stomach, and I remember waking up post-op on day one. I had a fever, a rapid pulse rate, and worsening pain. My surgeon's brain kicked in. I was taken back to the operating room multiple times for my leaking gastroesophageal anastomosis (where the esophagus was attached to the remainder of my stomach). This part is a bit hazy, but I knew enough to realize that I might die. I was told that my wife discussed the situation with my six-year-old daughter Maddi, preparing her for the possibility that Daddy might not come home. I had stents and drains. Eventually, I was well enough to leave and was discharged from the ICU. Multiple complications forced me to return to the hospital many times. Stent displacements, stricture dilation, esophageal perforation, and bile reflux. I experienced almost all the lovely complications one could have with this type of surgery.

I forgot to mention that while this was going on, I had returned to work. Patient rounds were interrupted multiple times so I could go to the bathroom and vomit bile. I had the pleasure of watching my family eat Thanksgiving dinner and then vomiting my birthday banana pudding. (I love carrot cake. My wife makes the absolute best carrot cake in the world, a true decadent pleasure. I had passed on it the previous year because I didn't think I could swallow it, and my daughter made me banana pudding instead.) More endoscopies and more surgery. A postoperative bowel obstruction required another abdominal exploration. I dealt with wound infection, intra-abdominal abscesses, four drains, and a lot of TPN (total parenteral nutrition) and IV antibiotics. I escaped on TPN on December 30, happy to be home and celebrate a late Christmas. I finally gained weight, and now I'm back doing what I love . . . not being the patient!

So what is the takeaway from this? Doctors need to remember that patients get scared. Surgery hurts. Be aware that the three to five minutes a day you spend with your patients doesn't do justice to their fears and concerns. Remember to listen to them when something new hurts. Don't assume they are a difficult pain-control problem. Assume they have a medical problem, and you need to figure it out. Listen to the families, the ones who stay at the bedside twenty-four hours a day. The ones who see the pain, the ones who witness nausea and vomiting, the ones who recognize subtle changes. Listen to the nurses who spend their days with your patients and see the same things. If they have questions, answer them. If they want to see you, see them. Listen to your patients with open ears, an open heart, and an open mind. Listen to their families.

BETWEEN A ROCK AND A HARD PLACE
By Yoram Klein, M.D.

Every young Israeli knows that a long journey overseas is a must after army service. The preferred destinations are either South America or Asia. These exotic places are also endemic regions for a few dangerous infectious diseases, so a series of vaccinations is mandatory before the beginning of the great adventure. Nella was a twenty-two-year-old officer in the Israeli Defense Forces (IDF) who had recently been discharged from her army duty. The detailed plans for her journey to South America were made, and the last thing to do before the flight was the vaccine series. The nurse at the geographic medicine center welcomed her warmly and started to prepare the vaccines. "When did you fall?" asked the nurse. Nella, surprised, said, "What are you talking about?" The nurse pointed at several blue marks on Nella's hands and thighs. Nella had not noticed the marks, so she decided to see her family doctor to be sure everything was okay before the trip. Well, everything was not okay. . . . Within a few days, Nella was diagnosed with acute leukemia, and the race to save her began. First, an aggressive chemotherapy protocol achieved remission of the disease. Simultaneously, an urgent search for a compatible bone marrow donor was started. Everybody was excited to hear that a donor was found, and a bone marrow transplantation was scheduled. In the meantime, Nella and the medical team decided to perform a fertility preservation procedure. In this operation, a piece of the ovary is removed and frozen for future use in case of infertility due to aggressive leukemia treatment. The operation went smoothly with no complications. But twenty-four hours after the operation, Nella started to feel excruciating abdominal pain, her blood pressure dropped, and a reddish secretion appeared in her pelvic drainage catheters. At that point, the gynecological team rushed her to the operating room and called me to assist them. A trauma surgeon can come in handy in these circumstances. We opened the abdomen and found that it was not bleeding. The issue was a severe case of acute pancreatitis—a known risk with aggressive chemotherapy. In most cases, acute pancreatitis is a mild disease. But rarely, this can be a devastating disease with necrosis of the pancreas and the fatty tissue around it. The most serious complication is an infection of the necrotic tissue, which requires invasive interventions and occasionally surgery, and sometimes the patient's abdomen is kept open for repeated operations to control the infection process. The most crucial aspect is that it takes time. A lot of time. Time that Nella could not afford to lose. Unfortunately, Murphy's law (if something can go wrong, it will) showed its ugly face, and two weeks later Nella was diagnosed with infected pancreatic necrosis. At that point, a race against time began. The first step in bone marrow transplantation is the destruction of the patient's native bone marrow, which meant Nella would be without an immune system. As a result, any minor infection could kill her. We had to eradicate the infection before the transplantation could take place. The transplantation had to be done before the effects of the previous chemotherapy subsided and leukemia reappeared. We were asking ourselves whether we should operate or wait. We consulted experts worldwide, but nobody had any experience with such a situation. We decided to stay with antibiotics and percutaneous drainage and not risk an operation that might leave Nella with an open abdomen for many weeks. The last chance for transplantation was approaching. Nella felt good, but the CT scan showed signs of a small area with infection. After endless discussions and hesitations, we decided to go ahead with the transplantation. Everybody was on their tiptoes, anxiously waiting for the outcome of the transplantation. A month later, the hematologist declared that Nella was off the hook . . . she had made a complete recovery.

Epilogue: In six years, if you find yourself in the emergency medicine department at Sheba Medical Center in Israel, you will notice a beautiful young blonde doctor with sparkling blue eyes. Nella started medical school a month ago.

AFTERWORD

*Men occasionally stumble over the truth, but most of them pick
themselves up and hurry off as if nothing had happened.*
WINSTON CHURCHILL (1874–1965)

Some "truths" about trauma surgery are contained in this book.
I hope I have facilitated a better understanding of who we
trauma surgeons are and what we do, and maybe a little of how we
think.

Unfortunately, most of the injuries that surgeons see today are
the same ones we saw when I started my training more than forty
years ago. The lack of changes among prevailing societal attitudes
toward seat belts, helmets, and driving while intoxicated, as well
as the plethora of weapons widely available in the United States,
are significant contributors to these injuries. In addition, the way
we treat injured patients and their outcomes is similar to treat-
ments of four decades ago. Why have advances in medical care
been so slow to occur in the trauma field? Despite injury being the
leading cause of lost productive years in the United States and of
the deaths of children and adults up to forty-four years of age,
trauma care remains woefully underfunded in terms of research.
Without dollars to support investigative efforts, there is simply no

way to perform quality studies to advance the science and improve patient outcomes.

Providing care to the injured and critically ill can be a daunting task, like fighting Mother Nature. We in the field have a lot of hope, but change is slow, and it can be frustrating to work in a "Groundhog Day" scenario, day after day, year after year. So the trauma team must be composed of optimists who rise each morning to fight the unchanging onslaught of injured people who fill our trauma centers. Unless there are changes in societal norms or better enforcement of laws, many of the injuries we see will continue to be unavoidable. One particularly problematic area for the trauma field is the seeming omnipresence of military-style weapons (estimated at over twenty million in the United States today, or about one for every sixteen Americans). Civilians owning rifles designed for combat is as logical as having 50-caliber machine guns or rocket launchers mounted on the roofs of our vehicles. One would hope that the continued rash of mass killings (647 in 2022 alone) will lead to some improved gun safety measures and eliminate this class of weapons for the general public. Ultimately, most of what we care for in trauma seems preventable.

Trauma surgery is certainly a challenging career, but the rewards are immense. The most gratifying aspect of my life as an academic trauma surgeon has been participating in the development of so many fine surgeons, many of whom now run their own excellent programs. I always considered them my oldest sons and daughters and have been so proud to see them evolve into leaders in the field. The educational environment in surgery is, in fact, quite nurturing and collaborative, and I learn something from each of my chief residents and fellows. Decades ago, I was invited by a former fellow (who is now a surgical residency program director) to be a visiting professor at a superb program thousands of miles away. During "professor rounds," while we were seeing some complex patients in the ICU, the residents were giggling. I asked what I had said that was so amusing. They responded that now they knew the origin of some of the expressions they had been hearing. Apparently, my words were repeated to them often by my former trainee.

So when most of your old fellows are now full professors, what does that make you? A dinosaur! Recently, after many decades in the field, I was asked when I planned to retire. Previously, I had always responded that I had no intention of retiring for many years. I hoped to continue to teach, perform research, and help with clinical care for a long time, assuming I could function at a high level. I still enjoy mentoring students, residents, and young faculty to be the best clinicians and academicians they can be. I used to say to the senior surgeons in my department, "You can die, but you're not allowed to retire." Why? Because we need their wisdom and their experience. There is simply no substitute for experience in the field of surgery. Any area of surgery. As my father used to say, "Any monkey can operate." This is pretty much the truth, but it takes experience and knowledge to judge whom to operate on, when to operate, and what operation to perform.

Unlike any other surgical subspecialty, trauma call is in-house (meaning sleeping overnight in the hospital), and this can be taxing physically and mentally. No matter how light the workload is on a particular night, covering the hospital overnight wipes you out for the next day. The average trauma surgeon in the United States takes five or six night calls per month; that is about a third of their life occupied by night call and its aftereffects. As one gets older, it's much harder to recover, and a reduction in the number of night calls is generally desirable. Burnout is common. Unfortunately, there is no way to easily support your salary and expenses as a trauma surgeon without taking night calls, unless you develop a large, lucrative general surgical practice or obtain a huge research grant. Likewise, doing a large amount of ICU call coverage can be a major grind. It's no wonder that most folks consider trauma surgery a young person's profession.

I recently spoke with a senior surgeon who is very accomplished and well known in the field. He cannot wait to retire at sixty-five; he is exhausted and no longer wishes to provide clinical care. It is a shame to lose all that expertise. Academic surgeons are expected to take a full clinical load and still teach and generate research. In contrast, on the internal medicine service, academic faculty typically cover a clinical service for only one or two months a year. The rest of the year is devoted to academic pursuits like teaching and research. One of the gentlemen I trained with in the Jurassic period is now contemplating retirement. He is a superb cancer surgeon—one of the best. When he steps down, there is simply no one who will be able to replace him. It would be ideal if he could remain in a position to mentor younger faculty for years; this would have a tremendous impact on the quality of patient care. Unfortunately, there do not appear to be many viable funded positions for excellent, experienced (a.k.a. old) surgeons who wish to focus on mentorship, education, and research while minimizing their clinical responsibilities.

I have been blessed with a lot of energy and have so far avoided clinical burnout, but the profession certainly wears on one's personal life. It is particularly difficult to have any predictable social life. For example, you cannot engage in a sports activity like playing in a basketball league or a weekly tennis game, and you can't regularly commit to any cultural event with your constantly varying schedule. The joys of helping people and aiding in the development of surgical trainees must be balanced against the impact the work has on your personal life.

Most trauma surgeons retire when they simply cannot tolerate the night call, the grind of ICU coverage, and the challenges of complex cases at inconvenient times. For me, the decision to retire will depend on how long I can endure the heavy workload and the medical politics that can make today's work environment particularly unpleasant. I am resisting this notion, as I feel that, like many senior, experienced surgeons, I still have a lot of wisdom left to offer.

ACKNOWLEDGMENTS

I would like to first acknowledge my wife, Miryame, who urged me to write down all the "wonderful" tales and information I had been inundating her with since we met. I realize it was partly to get me out of her hair as a "caged panther" during some downtime. But this was really her idea. I also truly appreciate her willingness to hear me read my chapters aloud to her, seemingly continuously for months on end. Her support was an act of true love. The continued love and challenge through the writing process of my grown-ass children, Sam, Liz, and Claudia, helped make the experience of writing worthwhile.

I also have to thank Janet Karmen profusely for all of her help. She was my first editor and was instrumental in putting together *All Bleeding Stops* in a form that is hopefully appealing to the public. Janet kept me honest and coherent and made sure I translated everything from medical speak to normal language. Thank you for all of your guidance, thoughts, and suggestions. And *no*, Jan, you have not contracted every disease in my book.

Big thanks to Randy Susan Meyers for voluntarily assisting me in understanding the process of publishing a book in the trade press and guiding me to various resources that made obtaining a literary agent possible. Writing a book for the public is much different from editing a surgical textbook for the academic press. Thank you to Dr. Pauline Chen, a former trainee, accomplished surgeon, and *New York Times* bestselling author, who helped me locate and approach a literary agent.

And, of course, I have to credit Don Fehr, my superb literary agent, for guiding me through the production of a book proposal and attracting a publisher. Don, it was painful but instructive. Finally, this book could not have been published without the help of Daniela Rapp and her associates at Mayo Clinic Press. This is new territory for me, and I truly appreciate your efforts to guide me on the path to success.

NOTES

CHAPTER 1. WHAT EXACTLY IS A TRAUMA SURGEON?

1. Stephen M. Cohn, Michelle A. Price, and C. Lizette Villarreal, "Trauma and Surgical Critical Care Workforce in the United States: A Severe Surgeon Shortage Appears Imminent," *Journal of the American College of Surgeons* 209, no. 4 (2009): 446–52.
2. Alexis Pozen and David M. Cutler, "Medical Spending Differences in the United States and Canada: The Role of Prices, Procedures, and Administrative Expenses," *Inquiry* 47, no. 2 (2010): 124–34.

CHAPTER 2. CONTROLLED CHAOS AT THE TRAUMA CENTER

1. "Deaths and Mortality," National Center for Health Statistics, https://www.cdc.gov/nchs/fastats/deaths.htm.

CHAPTER 3. CONSTRUCTING A SURGEON

1. Karl Y. Bilimoria et al., "National Cluster-Randomized Trial of Duty-Hour Flexibility in Surgical Training," *New England Journal of Medicine* 374, no. 8 (February 2016): 713–27, https://doi: 10.1056/NEJMoa1515724.
2. S. M. Cohn and S. T. Brower, eds., *General Surgery: Evidence-Based Practice* (Shelton, CT: PMPH, 2012); S. M. Cohn, M. O. Dolich, and K. Inaba, eds., *Acute Care Surgery and Trauma: Evidence-Based Practice*, 2nd ed. (Boca Raton, FL: CRC, 2016); S. M. Cohn and A. J. Feinstein, eds., *50 Landmark Papers in Trauma* (Boca Raton, FL: CRC, 2019); S. M. Cohn, S. O. Heard, and A. Lisbon, *50 Landmark Papers in Surgical Critical Care* (Boca Raton, FL: CRC, 2021); S. M. Cohn, ed., *Acute Care Surgery and Trauma: Evidence-Based Practice*, 3rd ed. (Boca Raton, FL: CRC, in press); S. M. Cohn and P. Rhee, eds., *50 Landmark Papers in Acute Care Surgery* (Boca Raton, FL: CRC, 2019).

CHAPTER 4. GENERALIST SURGEONS

1. Laura M. Stinton, Robert P. Myers, and Eldon A. Shaffer, "Epidemiology of Gallstones," *Gastroenterology Clinics of North America* 39, no. 2 (June 2010): 157–69.

CHAPTER 5. SAVING LIVES

1. Arthur L. Kellermann and Frederick P. Rivara, "Silencing the Silence on Gun Research," *Journal of the American Medical Association* 309, no. 6 (February 2013): 549–50, https://jamanetwork.com/journals/jama/fullarticle/1487470.
2. "NHTSA: Traffic Crashes Cost America $340 Billion in 2019," US Department of Transportation, January 10, 2023, https://www.nhtsa.gov/press-releases/traffic-crashes-cost-america-billions-2019.
3. Gentilello et al., "Alcohol Interventions in a Trauma Center as a Means of Reducing the Risk of Injury Recurrence," *Annals of Surgery* 230, no. 4 (October 1999): 473–80.
4. R. S. Thompson, F. P. Rivara, and D. C. Thompson, "A Case-Control Study of the Effectiveness of Bicycle Safety Helmets," *New England Journal of Medicine* 320, no. 21 (May 1989): 1361–67.

CHAPTER 6. DEALING WITH THE WORST INJURIES

1. Lee Shepherd, Ronan O'Carroll, and Eamonn Ferguson, "An International Comparison of Deceased and Living Organ Donation/Transplant Rates in Opt-in and Opt-out Systems: A Panel Study," *BMC Medicine* 12, no. 1 (September 2014): 131.
2. Matthew M. Grinsell, Sharon Showalter, Katherine A. Gordon, and Victoria F. Norwood, "Single Kidney and Sports Participation: Perception Versus Reality," *Pediatrics* 118, no. 3 (September 2006): 1019–27.
3. Michael R. Zemaitis, Lisa A. Foris, Richard A. Lopez, and Martin R. Huecker, *Electrical Injuries* (Treasure Island, FL: StatPearls, 2022).
4. John K. Bini, Stephen M. Cohn, Shirley M. Acosta, Marilyn J. McFarland, Mark T. Muir, and Joel M. Michalek, "Mortality, Mauling, and Maiming by Vicious Dogs," *Annals of Surgery*, no. 4 (April 2011): 791–97.

CHAPTER 7. MANAGING THE PUBLIC

1. Jian-Cang Zhou, Kong-Han Pan, Dao-Yang Zhou, San-Wei Zheng, Jian-Qing Zhu, Qiu-Ping Xu, and Chang-Liang Wang, "High Hospital Occupancy Is Associated with Increased Risk for Patients Boarding in the Emergency Department," *American Journal of Medicine* 125, no. 4 (April 2012): 416.e1–7.

2. M. A. Makary and M. Daniel, "Medical Error—The Third Leading Cause of Death in the US," *British Medical Journal* 353 (2016): 2139.

3. Elliott Bennett-Guerrero, Yue Zhao, and Sean M. O'Brien, "Variation in Use of Blood Transfusion in Coronary Artery Bypass Graft Surgery," *Journal of the American Medical Association* 304, no. 14 (October 2010): 1568–75.

4. Jeffrey L. Carson, Darrell J. Triulzi, and Paul M. Ness, "Indications for and Adverse Effect of Red-Cell Transfusion," *New England Journal of Medicine* 377 (2017): 1261–72.

5. John J. Como, Richard P. Dutton, Thomas M. Scalea, Bennett B. Edelman, and John R. Hess, "Blood Transfusion Rates in the Care of Acute Trauma," *Transfusion* 44, no. 6 (June 2004): 809–13.

6. Zachary J. Ward, Sara N. Bleich, Angie L. Cradock, Jessica L. Barrett, Catherine M. Giles, Chasmine Flax, Michael W. Long, and Steven Gortmaker, "Projected U.S. State-Level Prevalence of Adult Obesity and Severe Obesity," *New England Journal of Medicine* 381 (2019): 2440–50.

CHAPTER 8. PREVENTING INJURIES

1. Andrew K. Chang, Polly E. Bijur, Kevin G. Munjal, and E. John Gallagher, "Randomized Clinical Trial of Hydrocodone/Acetaminophen Versus Codeine/Acetaminophen in the Treatment of Acute Extremity Pain after Emergency Department Discharge," *Academic Emergency Medicine* 21, no. 3 (March 2014): 227–35.

2. Erin E. Krebs, Amy Gravely, Sean Nugent, Agnes C. Jensen, Beth DeRonne, Elizabeth S. Goldsmith, Kurt Kroenke, Matthew J. Blair, and Siamak Noorbaloochi, "Effect of Opioid vs. Nonopioid Medications on Pain-Related Function in Patients with Chronic Back Pain or Hip or Knee Osteoarthritis Pain: The SPACE Randomized Clinical Trial," *Journal of the American Medical Association* 319, no. 9 (2018): 872–82.

3. Ray W. Chang, Danielle M. Tompkins, and Stephen M. Cohn, "Are NSAIDs Safe? Assessing the Risk-Benefit Profile of Nonsteroidal Anti-inflammatory Drug Use in Postoperative Pain Management," *American Surgeon* 87, no. 6 (June 2021): 872–79.

4. Gili Kenet, Raphael Walden, Arieh Eldad, and Uri Martinowitz, "Treatment of Traumatic Bleeding with Recombinant Factor VIIa," *Lancet* 354, no. 9193 (November 1999): 1879.

CHAPTER 11. FRIENDS IN THE TRAUMA TRENCHES

1. Amin Hilman Zulkifli et al., "Takotsubo Cardiomyopathy: A Brief Review," *Journal of Medicine and Life* 13, no. 1 (2020): 3–7.

INDEX